HUMAN BODY REFLEX ZONE

quick lookups
bilingual anatomical
illustration of reflex zones
(english edition)

This book is one of four in the series;
Quick Reference Handbooks of Chinese Medicine

Editor
Guo Changqing
Yang Shujuan
Han Senning

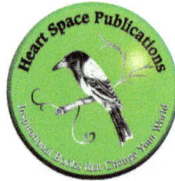

Published by

Heart Space Publications
PO Box 1085
Daylesford
Victoria
3460
Australia
Tel +61 450260348
www.heartspacebooks.com
pat@heartspacebooks.com

Whilst every care has been taken to check the accuracy of the information in this
book, the publisher cannot be held responsible for any errors, omissions or originality.
Published in 2021 at Melbourne

Medical information disclaimer – Although these practices have proven themselves
over eons, it is always a good idea to consult with your registered doctor or registered
health practitioner for any medical concerns. Always consider your medical officers
advice first. As the publisher of this manual, we make no warranties or claims, or
make any representations or warranties, express or implied as to the validity of these
practices.

ISBN 978-0-6489215-7-8

CONTENTS

Chapter IV Reflex zones of the hands 57

Human Body Reflex Zone Quick Lookup is an excellent book that introduces reflex zone therapy, including the major reflex zones of the scalp, face, ears, hands, feet and wrist-ankle acupuncture. These therapies have been used worldwide and been proven to be clinically effective in alleviating a variety of common symptoms. This book has concise and accurate descriptions of reflex points, accompanied by clear illustrations that allow the reader to easily locate reflex points. The information also includes the target symptoms for different reflex points. This book is not only helpful for clinical Chinese medical doctors, but also useful for medical school teachers and students. It is also suitable for Chinese medicine amateurs who can use this book as a guide to preventative treatment of conditions for themselves and their family.

Yueping Li, PhD of Chinese medicine
Australian registered Chinese Medical doctor and Acupuncturist

Introduction

The book is written by the experts and professors from Acupuncture-Moxibustion and the Tuina School of Beijing University of Chinese Medicine. They have selected the most commonly used and more effective reflex zone therapy for the book, and it is of high value of academics and clinical reference.

The book includes the reflex zone therapy of the scalp, face, ears, hands and feet, and mainly introduces the locations and indications of the reflex zones, with beautiful illustrations, so that it is characterized by conciseness and practicality, easiness for learning and remembering, and containing both texts and illustrations.

The book is mainly aimed at the clinical practitioners, teachers and researchers related to acupuncture, medical students, and TCM amateurs. It is a very practical pocket book for reflex zone therapy.

Preface

According to the theories of holographic biology, meridians and collaterals, and the nervous reflexes, reflex zone therapy is a natural healthcare technique that aims to activate the body's adaptive regulation through using certain methods, which stimulate the reflex zones in the corresponding holographic sections on the human body.

The reflex zone therapy has a long history in China. However, the records are scattered in different literatures and there is no proper formulated systematic theories.

At the beginning of the 20th century, Dr. William Fitzgerald, a pioneer of modern reflexology, published a book called *Zone Therapy* due to inspiration gathered from the Chinese acupuncture meridians theory.

By combining the theory of traditional Chinese medicine with the reflex zone therapy, Chinese medical practitioners gradually enriched and completed the reflex zone therapy, establishing a series of reflex zone therapies including zones for the scalp, face and ears, etc.

Reflex zone therapy has the functions of improving blood circulation, promoting metabolism, regulating the endocrine system, enhancing immunity, and regulating the functions of organs, so effects of treating diseases as well as boosting health can be achieved. The features of the therapy are all natural and safe, has good efficacy, has simple manipulations, and is convenient and economical as well as practical.

This book is mainly dedicated to clinical practitioners, teachers and researchers, who have any relation to acupuncture, medical students, as well as TCM amateurs. This is a very practical "pocket book" for reflex zone therapy.

Methods of Locating Combination Points

Section 1
Finger-length Measurement

Finger measurement is a method of standard measurement, for the location of the acupuncture point, since the fingers are in proportion with the other parts of the body – that the length and width of the patient's fingers are taken.

1. Four-Finger Measurement

The width of the four fingers (index, middle, ring and little) placed together, taken at the level of the dorsal crease of the proximal interphalangeal joint of the middle finger measures 3 cun. Cun is the term for the measurement relative to the patient (see images below). This method is always used to locate the points in the abdomen, back and lower limbs.

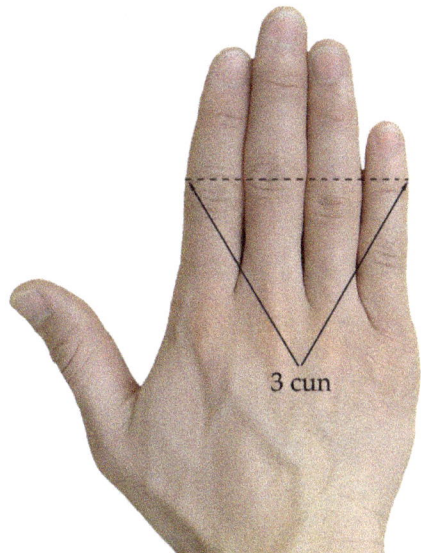

3 cun

2. Thumb Measurement

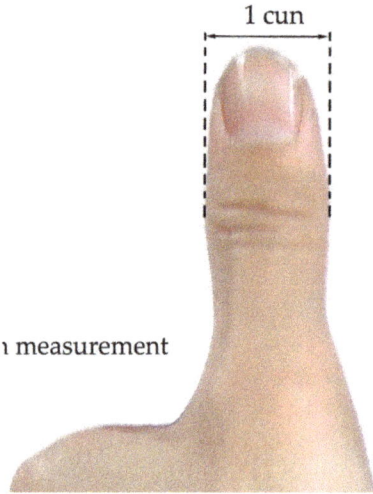

1 cun

Place the thumb straight. The width of the interphalangeal joint of the patient's thumb is 1 cun.

ı measurement

3. Middle Finger Measurement

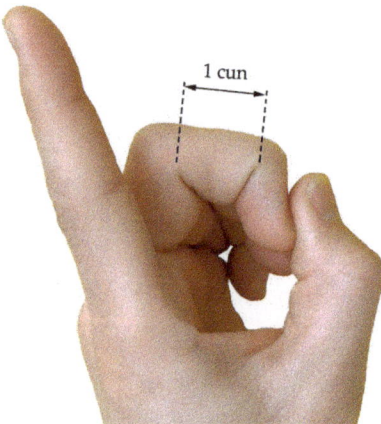

1 cun

When the patient's middle finger is flexed, the index finger is straight, and the end of the middle finger against the belly of the thumb, forming a ring. The width between the two medial ends of the creases of the interphalangeal joints is 1 cun. This method is suitable for limbs and transverse measurement of the dorsal.

Section 2
Bone-Length Measurement

The commonly used modern method of orientation of "bony degree" is based on Ling Shu (superior pivot), and in the long-term medical practice after modification and supplement, see the table below for details.

Standard for Bone-Length Measurement

Body Part	Area between two points on the body	Length in cun	
Head	From the midpoint of the anterior hairline to the midpoint of the posterior hairline	12 cun	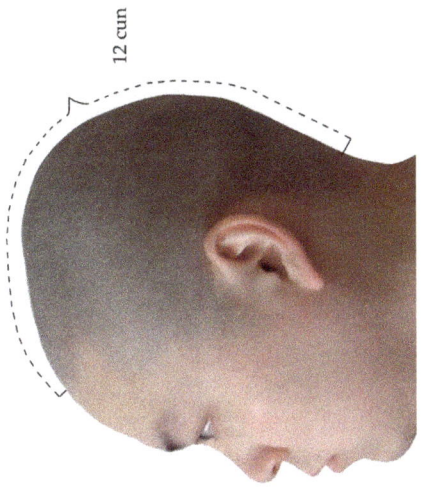

12 cun

Head	Between the corners of the forehead ST 8.	9 cun
Head	Between the two mastoid processes	9 cun
Chest and Abdomen	From the suprasternal fossa to the sterno-costal angle	9 cun
	From the sternocostal angle to the center of the umbilicus	8 cun
	From the center of the umbilicus to the upper of symphysis pubis	5 cun
	Between the two nipples	8 cun

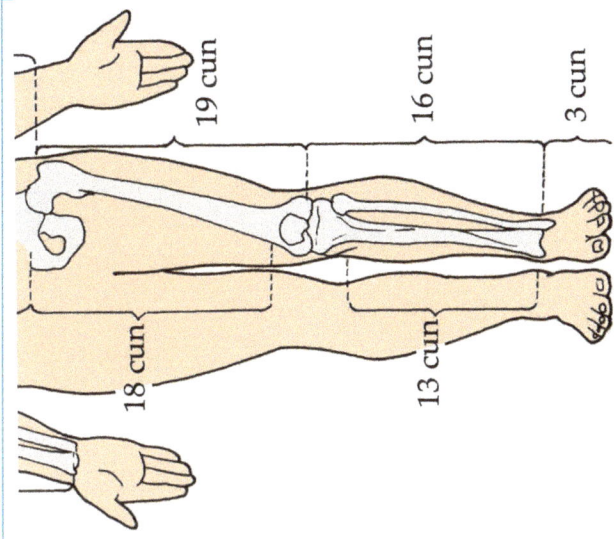

Lateral side of the trunk	From the tip of the axillary fossa to the tip of the 11th rib.	12 cun
	From the tip of the 11th rib to the prominence of the great trochanter	9 cun
Upper Limbs	From the end of the axillary fold to the transverse cubital crease	9 cun
	From the transverse cubital crease to the transverse wrist crease	12 cun
Lower Limbs	From the level of the border of symphysis pubis to the medial epicondyle of the femur	18 cun
	From the lower border of the medial condyle of tibia to the tip of medial malleolus	13 cun
	From the prominence of the great trochanter to the middle of patella	19 cun
	From the center of patella to the tip of lateral malleolus	16 cun
	From the tip of lateral malleolus to the sole.	3 cun

CHAPTER I

Reflex zones of the scalp

Reflex zones therapy of the scalp is a method of acupuncture that applies to specific areas of the scalp to treat a specific disease. Also known as acupuncture, scalp acupuncture, and or scalp penetration acupuncture therapy. Scalp reflex zone therapy of the treatment line is founded on TCM theory, developed in accordance with the principle of "fixed points by District, joint hole crossed meridian line". It divides the scalp into four districts, and 14 lines. These are;

1. Midcourt line of forehead

Position	in the middle of the forehead hairline, the spontaneous interpersonal GV 24 from the downward stab 1-cun (with body, the same below).
Indications	the mind of disease, head, nose, tongue, eyes, throat disease.

2. 1 wire next to midcourt line (acupoints in head are connected, and thus they are called wire)

Position	in the forehead, outside the midcourt line of forehead, straight eye angles (head, the inner canthus), from 0.5 cun at the spontaneous interpersonal meichong points insert one cun down.
Indications	disease of the lung, heart, etc..

3. 2 wire next to 1-wire

Position	in the forehead, next to 1-wire, faced straight to the pupil, from 0.5 cun at the spontaneous interpersonal toulinqi points(Gb-15) insert one cun down.
Indications	in the focus of the spleen, stomach, liver, and gall bladder disease.

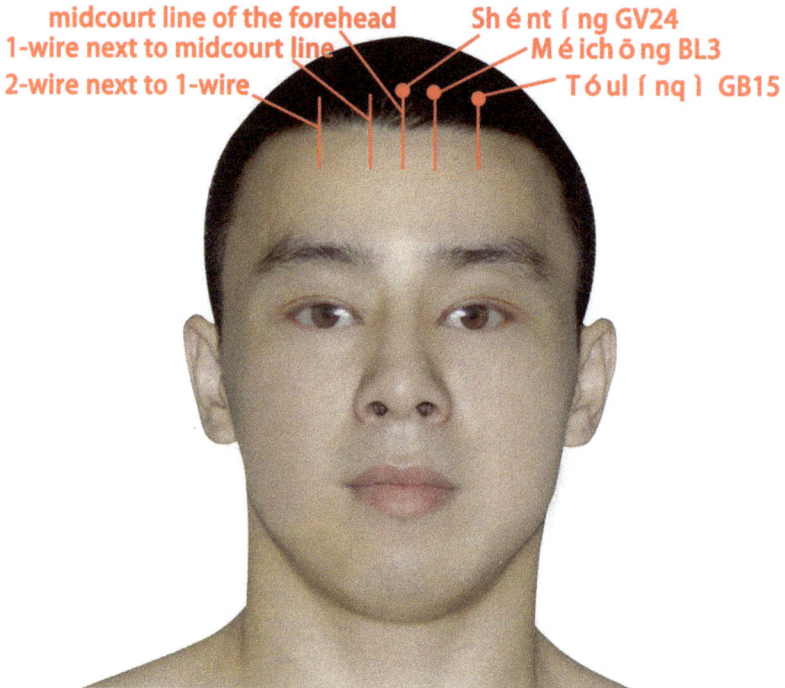

Figure 1-1 midcourt line of the forehead 2—wire next to 1-wire

4. 3-wire next to 2-wire

Position	in the forehead, located next to 2-wire, faced straight to outer corner of the eyes, inside 0.75-cun of the touwei points (between benshen points, Gb 13 and touwei points, ST 8) from 0.5 cun at the spontaneous interpersonal, insert one cun down.
Indications	the next focus of disease of the kidney, bladder.

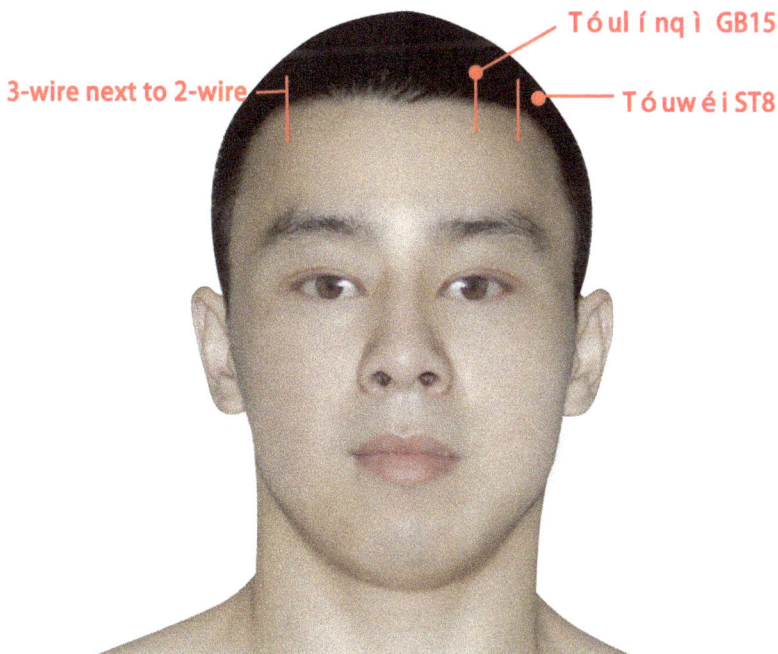

Figure 1-2 3-wire next to 2-wire

5. Top of the center line

Position	in the top of the head, located around the midline, from Baihui (Du 20) to qianding (Du 21) point.
Indications	the waist, legs and foot diseases.

6. 1-wire next to the center line

Position	in the top of the head, outside the top of the center line, with 1.5 cun apart, from the tongtian (Bl 7) point along the meridian insert 1.5 cun backwards.
Indications	the waist, legs, and foot disease, such as lower limb paralysis, numbness, pain.

7. 2-wire next to 1-wire

Position	on the top of the head outside 1-wire, with 0.75 cun apart, from zhengying (Gb 17) point along the meridian insert 1.5 cun backwards.
Indications	the shoulders, arms and hands diseases.

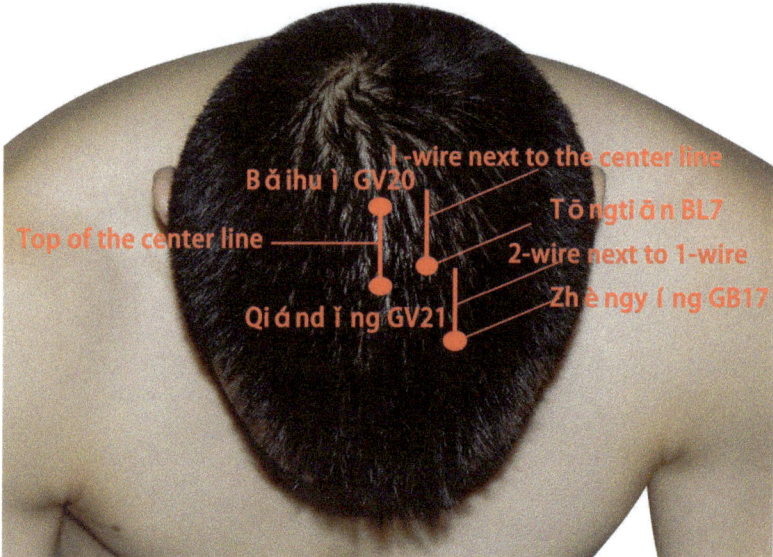

Figure 1-3 Top of the center line—2-wire next to l -wire

8. Top temporal forward slash

Position	on the side of the head, from top of the head to the head temporal region, the connection line between qian-shencong (EX-HNI) and xuanli (GB 6) points.
Indications	motor dysfunction symptoms such as paralysis, etc. The whole line can be divided into five equal portions, the upper 1/5 rule lower limb paralysis, the middle 2/5 rule upper limb paralysis, the lower 2/5 rule facial paralysis, motor aphasia, salivation.

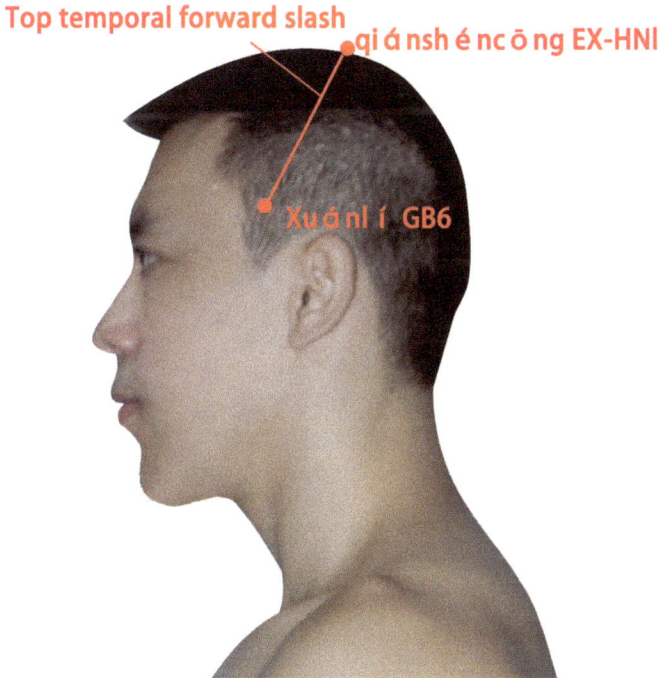

Top temporal forward slash

qiánshéncōng EX-HNI

Xuánlí GB6

Figure 1-4 Top temporal forward slash

9. Top temporal after the slash

Position	at the side of the head, from top of the head to the head temporal region, after the top temporal **foruard** slash, with 1.5-cun apart, that is, the connection line between Baihui (GV 20) and Qubin (GB 7) points.
Indications	sensory dysfunction diseases, such as pain, numbness, itching, etc. The upper 1/5 rule lower limb paresthesia, the middle 2/5 rule upper limb paresthesia, the lower 2/5 rule head facial paresthesia.

10. Temporal frontline

Position	inside the hair on the temples of the head, the connection line between hanyan (GB4) and xuanli (GB 6) points.
Indications	migraine, aphasia, peripheral facial paralysis and Oral Pathology psychosis.

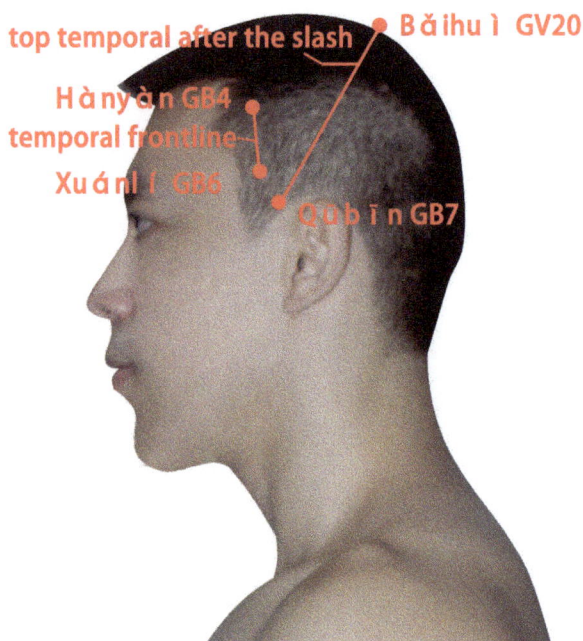

Figure 1-5 top temporal after the slash—temporal frontline

11. Temporal line

Position	in the region of temporal head, the connection line between shuaigu (Gb8) and qubin (Gb7) points.
Indications	migraine headaches, vertigo, tinnitus, deafness.

12. Pillow midline

Position	it is located at the occipital head, the perpendicular line upright the external occipital protuberance, the connection line between qiangjian (Du18) and naohu (Du17) points.
Indications	eye disease, lumbar pain.

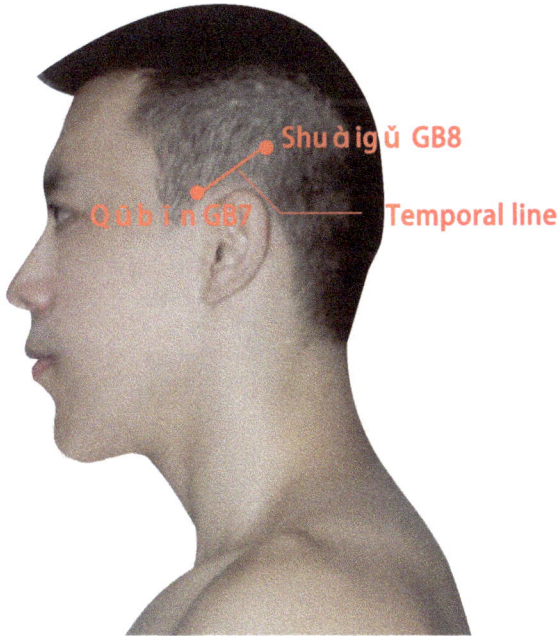

Figure 1-6 Temporal line

13. Side line on pillow

Position	it is located at the occipital head with pillow midline parallel led, the straight line which is 0.5 cun away from pillow midline.
Indications	the same with pillow midline.

14. Side line under pillow

Position	at the occipital head, the perpendicular line which is 2-cun-long below the external occipital protuberance from yuzhen (Bl9) to tianzhu (Bl10) points.
Indications	symptoms of balance disorders caused by cerebella disease, back headaches.

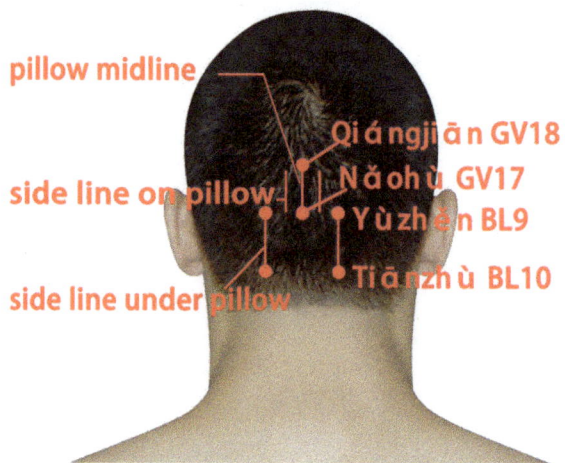

pillow midline

Qiángjiān GV18

Nǎohù GV17

side line on pillow

Yùzhěn BL9

Tiānzhù BL10

side line under pillow

Figure 1-7　Pillow midline—side line under pillow

　Human Body Reflex Zone

CHAPTER II

Reflex zones of the face

Facial reflex zone therapy is to stimulate specific reflex zones of the face, to treat a variety of diseases. Reflex zones of the face amounts of 7 central reflex zones; such as forehead, nose and upper lip median. Also, it includes 17 pairs of reflex zones, which are next to the nose, eyes, mouth, malar and cheek.

1. The first

Position	at the center point of forehead.
Indications	headache and dizziness.

2. Lung point (Yintang)

Position	at the midpoint of the connection line inside the two eyebrows.
Indications	cough and chest tightness.

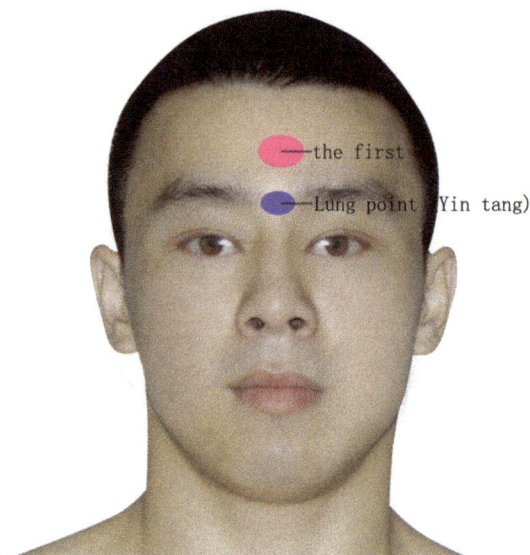

Figure 2-1 the first—Lung point (Yintang, EM2)

3. Sore throat

Position	at the midpoint of the connection line between the first and lung point.
Indications	throat, swelling.

4. Heart (foot)

Position	at the point of the nose bone, the midpoint between two inner canthus.
Indications	palpitations, insomnia.

5. Ying milk

Position	at the midpoint between heart point and inner canthus.
Indications	Reduced breast milk flow.

6. Liver

Position	connected with nasal cartilage under the nose bone, which is below the heart point.
Indications	two hypochondriac pain, chest tightness.

7. Gallbladder

Position	located on both sides of the liver point, below two inner canthus, under the nose bone margin.
Indications	nausea, vomiting.

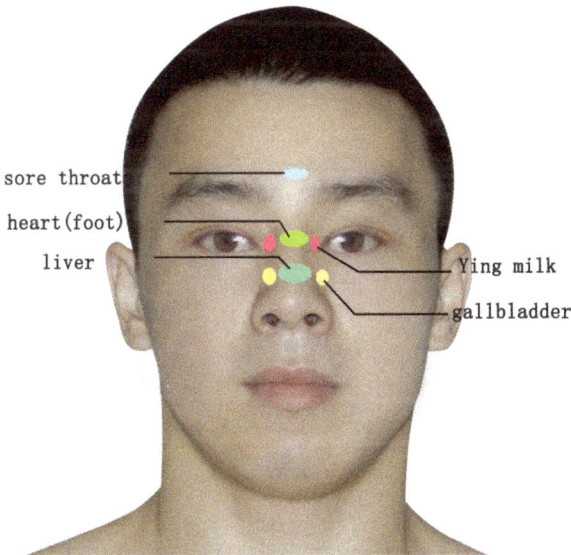

Figure 2-2 sore throat—gall bladder

8. Spleen (suliao)

Position	at the top of nose
Indications	reduced appetite, anorexia.

9. Bladder & Uterus

Position	located at the midpoint of renzhong (Du26) gap.
Indications	dysmenorrhea.

10. Inner unit

Position	near dicang point (ST4), 0.5 cun next to the corner of the mouth, at the anastomotic between upper and lower lip line.
Indications	vastus pain.

11. Stomach

Position	on both sides of spleen point in the center of alar.
Indications	stomach pain.

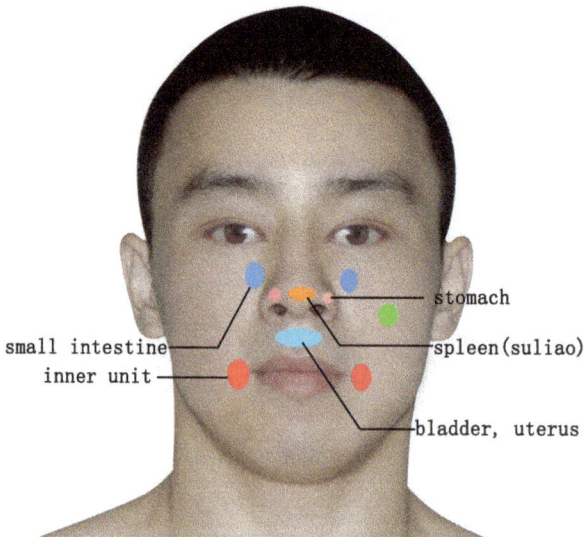

Figure 2-3 spleen (suliao)—stomach

12. Small intestine

Position	located outside the midpoint of the connection between gall bladder point and stomach point.
Indications	diarrhea.

13. Large intestine

Position	it is located under the outer canthus, under the cheek-bones.
Indications	constipation, abdominal pain, and diarrhea.

14. Shoulder

Position	located under the outer canthus, outside the gallbladder point.
Indications	shoulder – arm pain, flexor and extensor adversely.

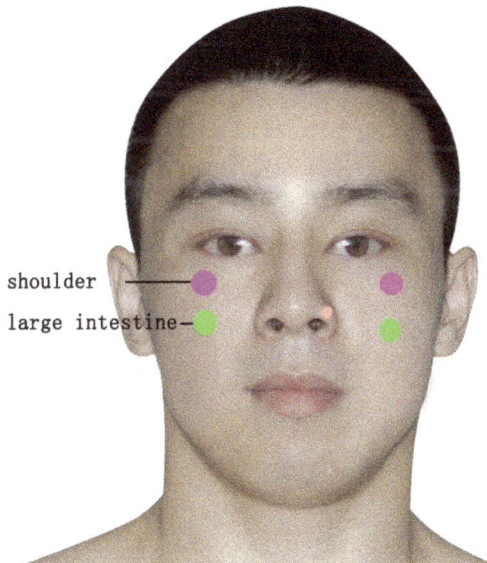

Figure 2-4 large intestine shoulder

15. Arm

Position	at the crossing point between the position behind arm point and the position upright xiaguan (ST7) point.
Indications	shoulder – arm pain and swelling.

16. Heading mission

Position	located below the arm point, the lower edge of zygomatic arch.
Indications	hand swelling and pain.

17. Back (Tinggong, SI 19)

Position	1 cun behind the center of cheer.
Indications	lumbar back pain.

18. Kidney

Position	at the crossing point between the line that parallels to alae nasi and the perpendicular line under taiyang point (EM5).
Indications	liguria, urinary pain, urinary frequency.

19. Umbilical

Position	located 0.3 cun under the kidney point.
Indications	abdominal pain.

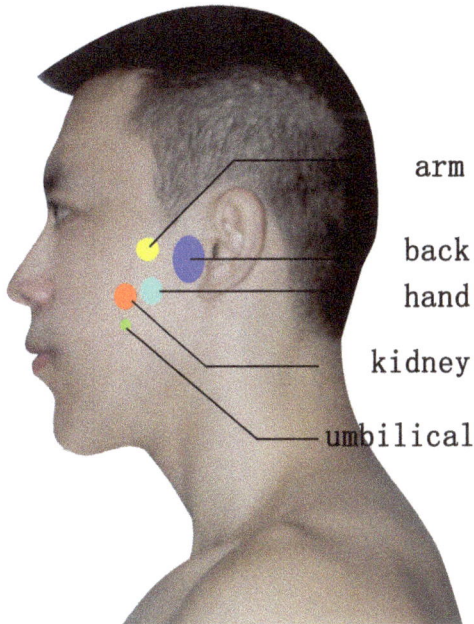

arm

back

hand

kidney

umbilical

Figure 2-5 arm—umbilical

20. Unit

Position	the crossing point that is, the upper one-third on the connection line between lobulus auriculae and mandibular angle.
Indications	thigh sprain.

21. Knee

Position	located at the crossing point, that is, the lower one-third on the connection line between lobulus auriculae and mandibular angle.
Indications	patellar and knee pain and swelling.

22. Knee and patellar (jiache, ST6)

Position	it is located in the hollow upright of the mandibular angle.
Indications	knee joint injury.

23. Tibia

Position	located in front of the mandible angle, the end of the mandible bone.
Indications	ankle sprain, muscle spasms.

24. Foot

Position	located in front of tibia point, under the outer acanthus, the upper edge of the mandible bone.
Indications	foot pain and swelling.

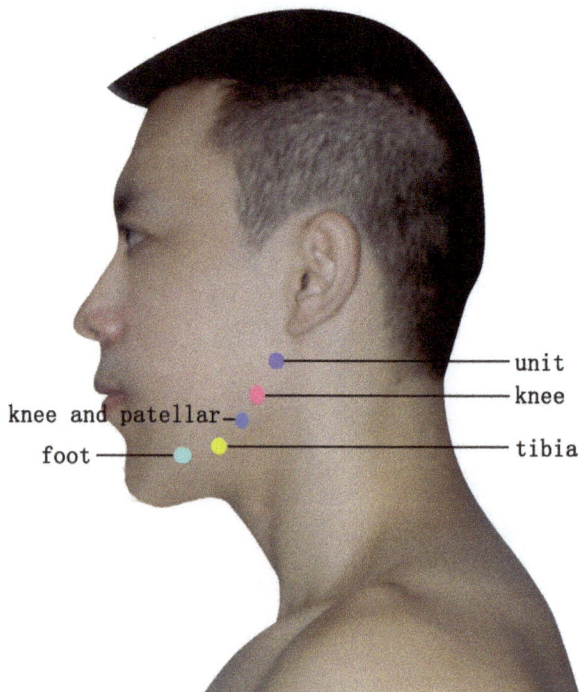

Figure 2-6 unit—foot

CHAPTER III

Reflex zones of the ears

Reflex zones of the ears therapy (Auricular acupuncture points) is a method to prevent and treat diseases by applying needles or other tools to stimulate the points of the ears. In order to make it convenient to research and communicate, China was authorized by the World Health Organization Regional Office for Western Pacific to formulate the International Standard of Auricular Points (ISPA).

Part I   Eight Points on the Helix

1. Ear center

Position	on the crus of the helix.
Indications	hiccups, urticaria, cutaneous pruritus, infantile enuresis, hemoptosis.

2. Rectum

Position	on the helix to the notch superior to the tragus and level with Large Intestine.
Indications	constipation, diarrhea, prolapse of the anus, hemorrhoids.

3. Urethra

Position	on the helix superior to Rectum, and level with bladder.
Indications	frequent, urgent or painful urination, urinary retention.

4. External genitals

Position	on the helix superior to urethra, and level with sympathetic nerve.
Indications	testitis, epididymitis, vulvar or scrotal pruritus.

5. Anus

Position	on the helix level with the anterior border of the superior crus of the antihelix.
Indications	hemorrhoids, anal fissure.

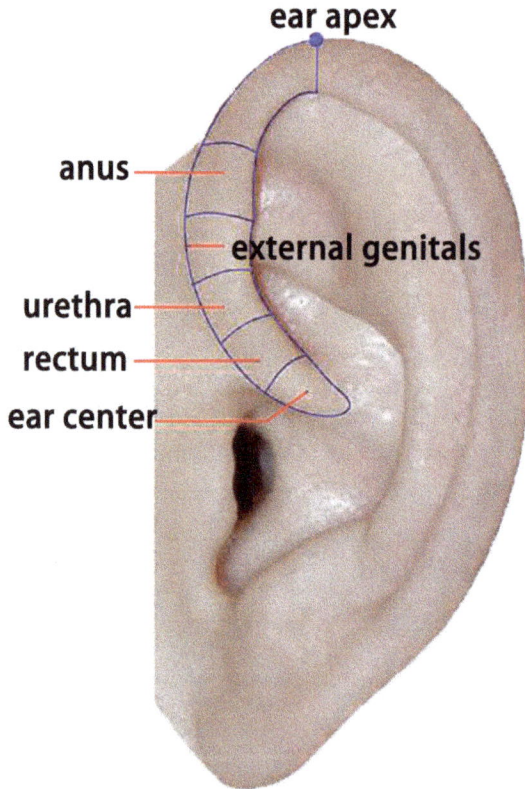

Figure 3-1 ear center—anus

6. Ear apex

Position	on the helix level with the posterior to the superior crus of the antihelix.
Indications	fever, hypertension, acute conjunctivitis

7. Node

Position	at the tubercle of the helix.
Indications	dizziness, headache, hypertension.

8. Helix 1, helix 2, helix 3 & helix 4

Position	on the helix, from the tubercle of the helix to the notch of the helix-lobe is separated into 4 equal sections. The four points are, from top to bottom, helix 1, helix 2, helix 3, & helix 4.
Indications	tonsillitis, upper respiratory tract infection, fever.

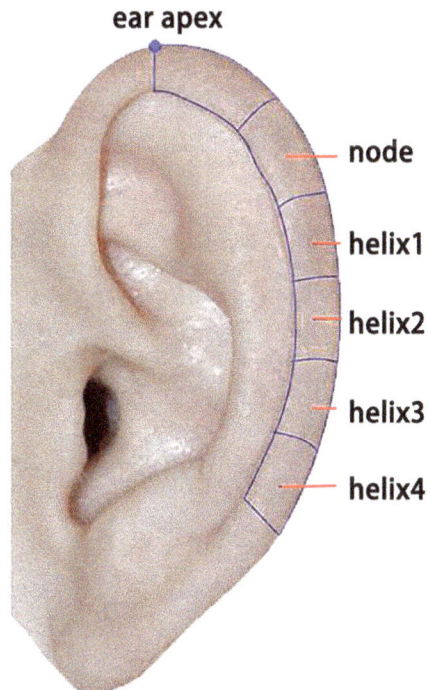

Figure 3-2 ear apex— helix 1, helix 2, helix 3 & helix 4

Part II   Six points in the scapha

1. Fingers

Position	the scaphoid fossa is divided into six equal parts, the first part, from top to bottom, is finger.
Indications	paronychia, pain and numbness of the fingers.

2. Wind stream

Position	between Fingers and Wrist.
Indications	urticaria, cutaneous pruritus, allergic rhinitis.

3. Wrist

Position	on the second part from the top of the scaphoid fossa.
Indications	wrist pain.

4. Elbow

Position	on the third part from the top of the scaphoid fossa.
Indications	tennis elbow, elbow pain.

5. Shoulder

Position	on the fourth and fifth part from the top of the scaphoid fossa.
Indications	scapulohumeral periarthritis, shoulder pain.

6. Clavicle

Position	on the sixth part from the top of the scaphoid fossa.
Indications	scapulohumeral periarthritis.

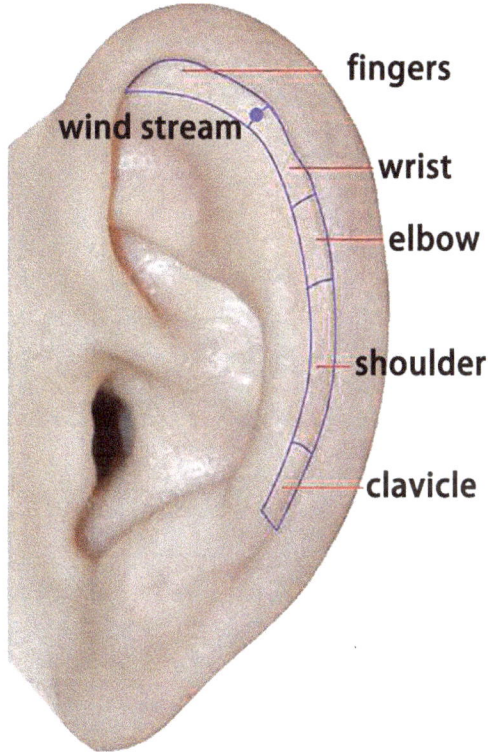

Figure3-3 fingers—clavicle

Part III   Five points in the superior antihelix crus

1. Toes

Position	on the posterior/superior area of the superior crus of the antihelix, close to the apex.
Indications	paronychia, pain in the toes.

2. Heel

Position	on the anterior superior of the superior crus of the antihelix, close to the upper portion of the triangular fossa.
Indications	heel pain.

3. Ankle

Position	between Heel and Knee.
Indications	strain of the ankle joint.

4. Knee

Position	on the middle one third of the superior crus of the antihelix.
Indications	swelling and pain of the knee joint.

5. Hip

Position	located on the lower one third of the superior antihelix crus.
Indications	pain of the hip joint, sciatica.

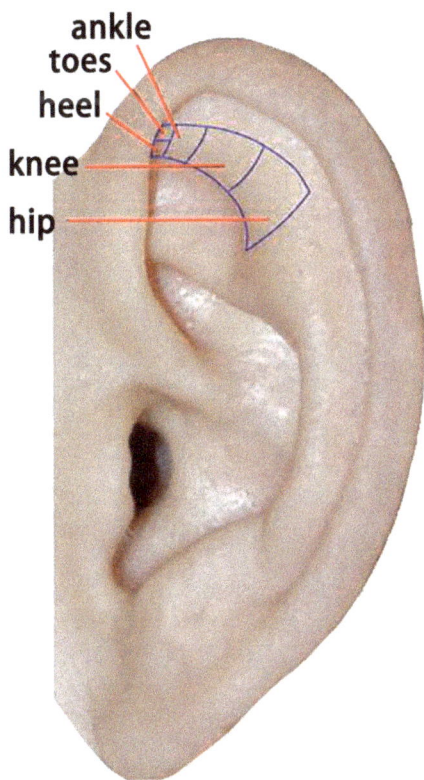

Figure 3-4 toes—hip

Part IV   Three points in the inferior antihelix crus

1. Gluteus

Position	on the posterior one third of the inferior crus of the antihelix.
Indications	sciatica, gluteal fasciitis.

2. Sciatic nerve

Position	on the anterior two-third of the inferior crus of the antihelix.
Indications	sciatica.

3. Sympathetic nerve

Position	on the juncture of the terminal of the inferior crus of the antihelix and the helix.
Indications	gastrointestinal spasm, angina pectoris, biliary colic, ureterolithiasis, functional disturbance of the autonomic nervous system.

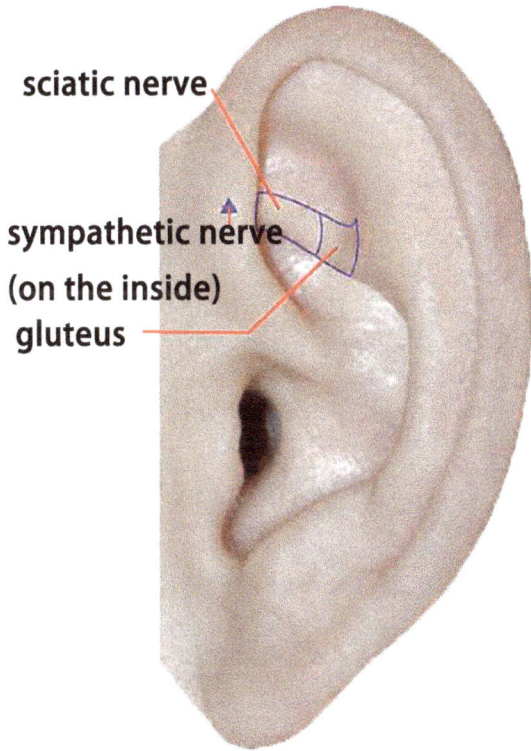

Figure 3-5 gluteus—sympathetic nerve

Part V   Six points in the body of the antihelix

1. Cervical vertebrae

Position	the body of the antihelix (the area between the notch separating the antitragus and the antihelix, and the origin of the superior and inferior crus of the antihelix) is divided into 5 parts. It is located on the lower one-fifth of the antihelix.
Indications	stiff neck, cervical spondylopathy.

2. Thoracic vertebrae

Position	on the middle 2/5th of the body of the antihelix.
Indications	chest pain, premenstrual swelling of the breasts, mastitis, postpartum lactation.

3. Lumbosacral vertebrae

Position	on the lower 2/5th of the body of the antihelix.
Indications	pain in the lumbosacral region.

4. Neck

Position	on the border of the concha anterior to the Cervical Vertebrae.
Indications	stiff neck, neck swelling and pain.

5. Chest

Position	on the border of the concha anterior to the Thoracic Vertebrae.
Indications	pain in the chest or hypochondriac region, feeling fullness in the chest, mastitis.

6. Abdomen

Position	on the border of the concha anterior to the Lumbosacral Vertebrae.
Indications	abdominal pain, bloating, diarrhea, acute lumbar sprain.

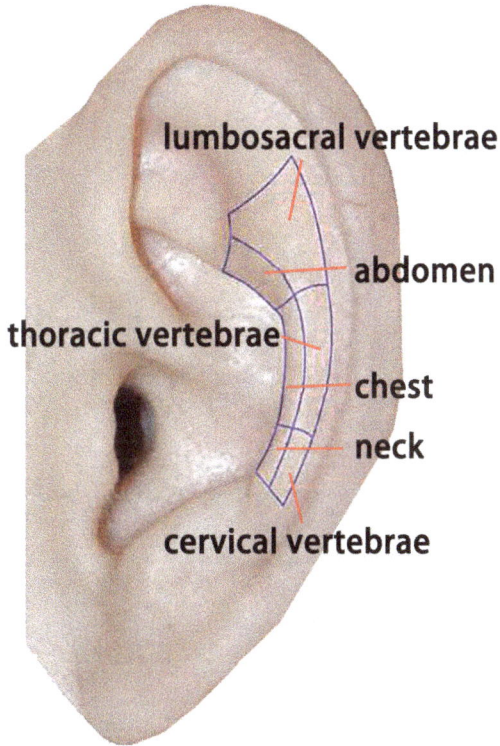

Figure 3-6 cervical vertebra—abdomen

Part VI   Five points on the triangular fossa

1. Shenmen (HT 7)

Position	on the triangular fossa superior to the origin of the superior and inferior crus of the antihelix.
Indications	palpitations, excessive dreaming, pain, withdrawal syndrome.

2. Pelvis

Position	on the triangular fossa inferior to the origin of the superior and inferior crus of the antihelix.
Indications	pelvis inflammation.

3. Middle triangular fossa

Position	on the middle 1/3th of the triangular fossa.
Indications	asthma.

4. Internal genitals

Position	on the anterior 1/3 of the triangular fossa.
Indications	dysmenorrhea, irregular menstruation, leukorrhagia, dysfunctional uterine bleeding, seminal emission, premature ejaculation.

5. Superior triangular fossa

Position	anterior/superior to the triangular fossa.
Indications	hypertension.

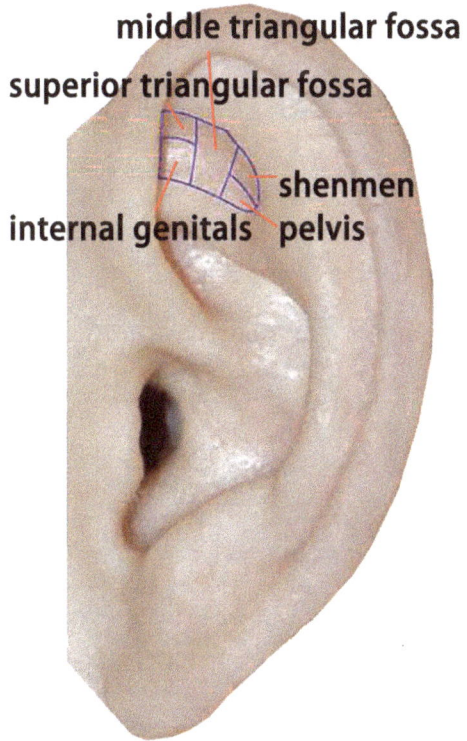

Figure 3-7 Shenmen—superior triangular fossa

Part VII Nine points on the tragus

1. Upper tragus

Position	on the upper 1/2 of the external surface of the tragus.
Indications	pharyngitis, simple obesity.

2. Lower tragus

Position	in the lower 1/2 of the external surface of the tragus.
Indications	rhinitis, obesity.

3. External ear

Position	anterior to the notch of the tragus close to helix.
Indications	external auditory canal, otitis media, tinnitus.

4. External nose

Position	slightly anterior to the midpoint of the external surface of the tragus.
Indications	nasal vestibulitis, rhinitis.

5. Apex of tragus

Position	on the top of the upper eminence of the tragus.
Indications	fever, toothache.

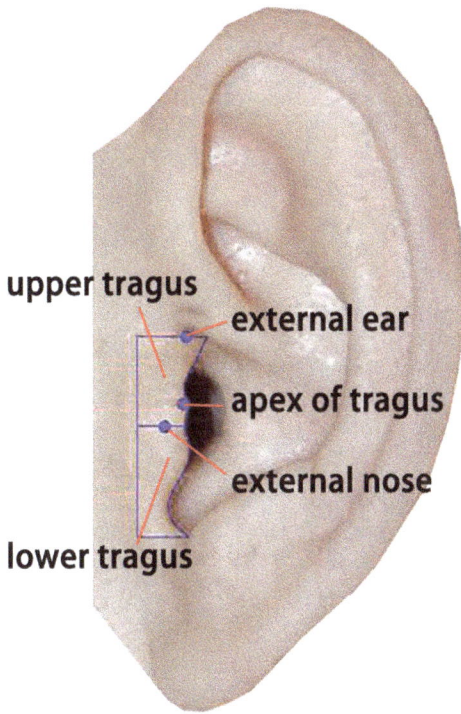

Figure 3-8 upper tragus—apex of tragus

6. Adrenal gland

Position	on the top of the lower eminence of the tragus.
Indications	hypotension, rheumatoid arthritis, mumps, intermittent malaria, vertigo caused by streptomycin poisoning.

7. Anterior intertragic notch

Position	located at the lowest part of the front surface of the intertragic notch on the inferior edge of TG2.
Indications	eye disease.

8. Pharynx and larynx

Position	on the upper 1/2 of the internal side of the tragus.
Indications	hoarseness, pharyngitis, tonsillitis.

9. Internal nose

Position	on the lower 1/2 of the internal side of the tragus.
Indications	rhinitis, paranasal sinusitis, epistaxis.

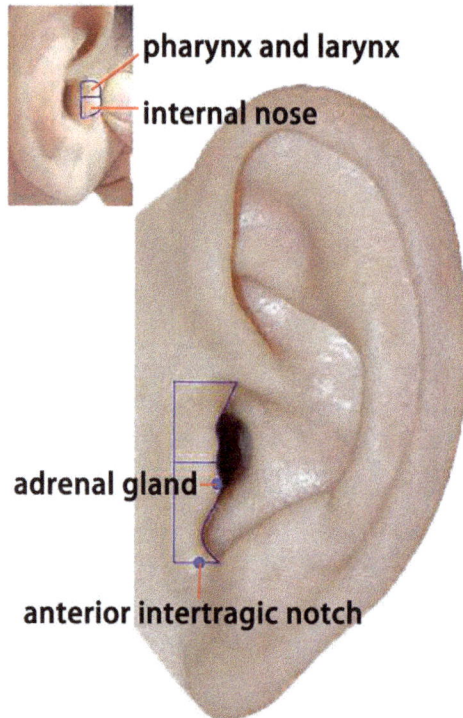

Figure 3-9 adrenal gland—internal nose

Part VIII   Eight points on the antitragus

1. Apex of antitragus

Position	on the upper portion of the antitragus.
Indications	asthma, parotitis, cutaneous pruritus, testitis, epididymitis.

2. Central rim

Position	on the midpoint between Apex of Antitragus and the notch between the antitragus and the antihelix.
Indications	nocturnal enuresis, meniere's disease.

3. Occiput

Position	on the posterior/superior part of the external surface of the antitragus.
Indications	headache, dizziness, asthma, epilepsy, neurasthenia.

4. Temple

Position	on the middle part of the external surface of the antitragus.
Indications	migraine.

5. Forehead

Position	on the anterior/inferior part of the external surface of the antitragus.
Indications	headache, dizziness, insomnia, dreaminess.

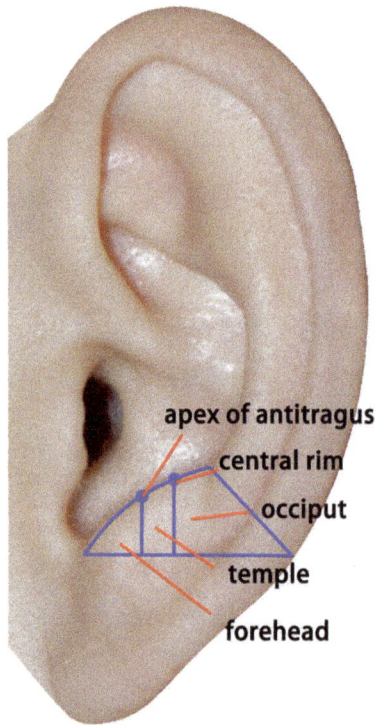

Figure 3-10 apex of antitragus—forehead

6. Posterior intertragicus

Position	on the inferior part of antitragus posterior to the anti-tragus notch on the lower edge of AT1.
Indications	eye disease.

7. Brain stem

Position	at the antihelix-antitragus notch at the juncture of AT3 and AT4.
Indications	headache, dizziness, pseudomyopia.

8. Subcortex

Position	on the internal side of the antitragus.
Indications	pain, intermittent malaria, neurasthenia, pseudomyopia.

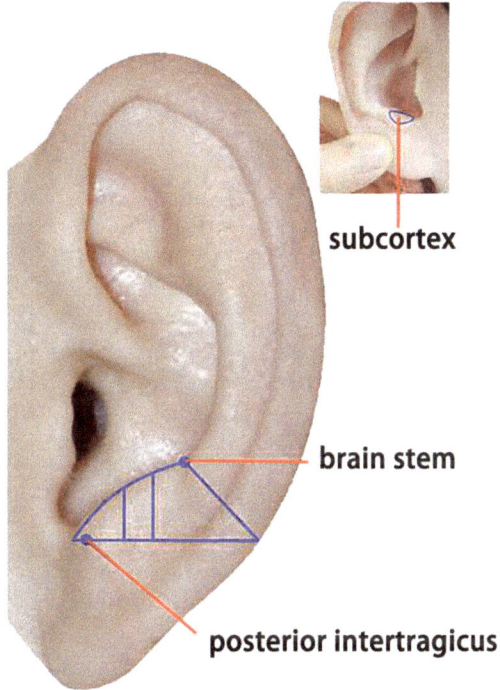

subcortex

brain stem

posterior intertragicus

Figure 3-11 posterior intertragicus—subcorte

Part IX   Eight points around the helix crus

1. Large intestine

Position	anterior to the superior of the crus of the helix.
Indications	diarrhea, constipation, dysentery, cough, acne.

2. Small intestine

Position	in the middle of the superior of the crus of the helix.
Indications	indigestion, abdominal distention, tachycardia, arrhythmia.

3. Appendix

Position	between Large intestine and Small intestine.
Indications	simple appendicitis, diarrhea.

4. Duodenum

Position	inferior to the superior of the crus of the helix.
Indications	duodenal ulcer, cholecystitis, gallstones, pylorospasm.

5. Stomach

Position	on the terminus of the crus of the helix.
Indications	stomach cramps, gastritis, stomach ulcers, insomnia, toothache, indigestion.

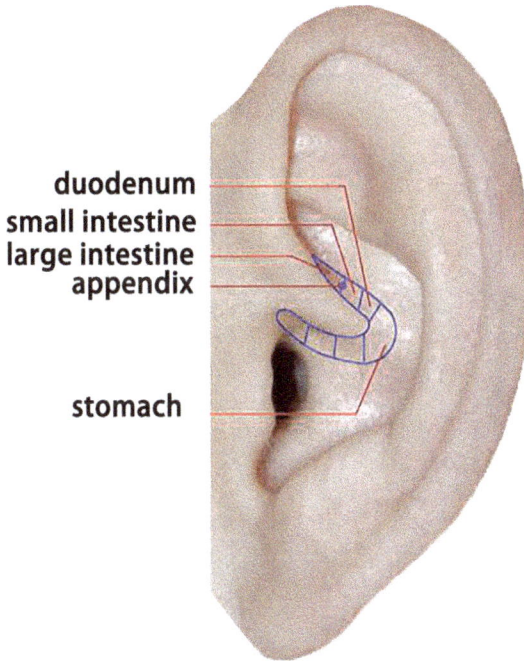

Figure 3-12 large intestine—stomach

6. Cardia

Position	on the posterior 1/3 of the inferior to the crus of the helix.
Indications	cardiospasm, neurogenic vomiting.

7. Esophagus

Position	in the middle 1/3 of the inferior to the crus of the helix.
Indications	esophagitis, esophagospasm, globus hystericus.

8. Mouth

Position	anterior 1/3 of the inferior to the crus of the helix.
Indications	facial paralysis, stomatitis, cholecystitis, gallstones, withdrawal syndrome.

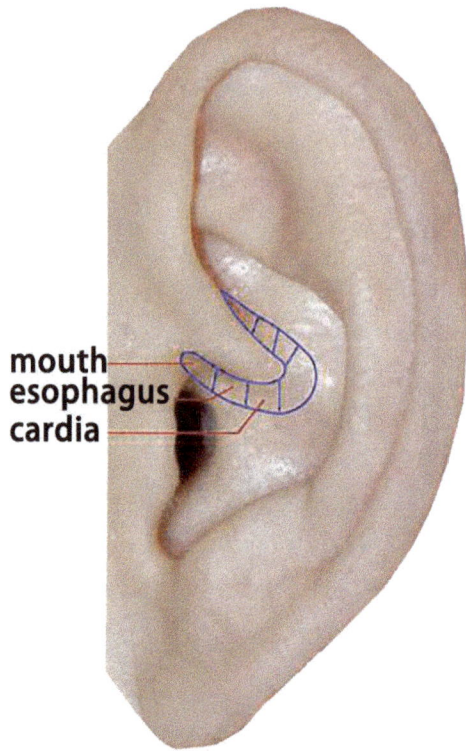

Figure 3-13 cardia—mouth

Part X   Six points on the cavum conchae

1. Heart

Position	on the center of the depression of the cavum conchae.
Indications	tachycardia, arrhythmia, angina pectoris, pulseless disease, neurasthenia, hysteria, stomatoglossitis.

2. Lung

Position	surrounding the middle of the depression of the cavum conchae.
Indications	cough, feeling of fullness in the chest, hoarseness, acne, cutaneous pruritus, urticaria, flat warts, constipation, withdrawal syndrome.

3. Trachea

Position	on the cavum conchae between the foramen of the external auditory canal and heart.
Indications	cough, asthma.

4. Spleen

Position	on the inferp/osterior part of the cavum conchae.
Indications	bloating, diarrhea, constipation, poor appetite, dysfunctional uterine bleeding, leukorrhagia, Meniere's disease.

5. Endocrine

Position	in the lower part of the cavum conchae close to the intertragus notch.
Indications	dysmenorrhea, irregular menstruation, menopausal syndrome, acne, intermittent malaria.

6. Triple energizer

Position	in the lower part of the cavum conchae superior to the Tragus.
Indications	constipation, bloating, pain in the lateral side of the upper limbs.

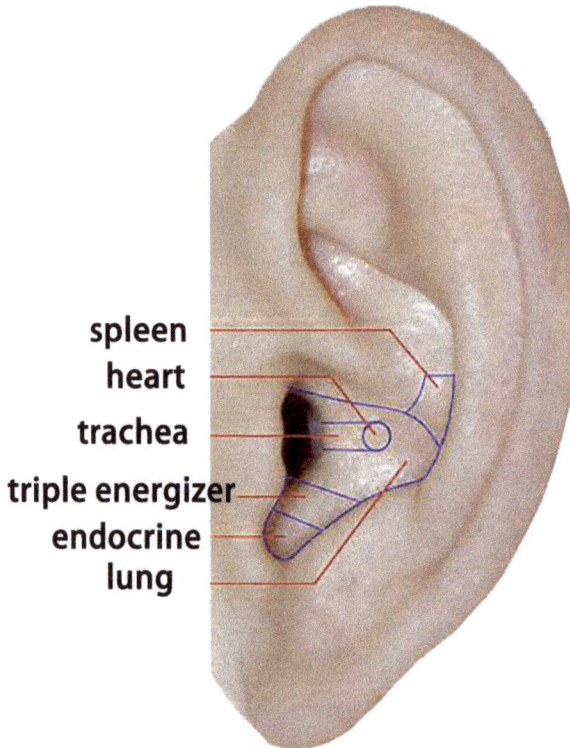

spleen
heart
trachea
triple energizer
endocrine
lung

Figure 3-14 heart—triple energizer

Part XI   Seven points in the cymba concha

1. Liver

Position	on the posterior inferior of the cymba concha.
Indications	pain in the chest and hypochondriac region, dizziness, premenstrual tension, irregular menstruation, menopausal syndrome, hypertension, pseudomyopia, simple glaucoma.

2. Pancreas and gallbladder

Position	between Liver and Kidney.
Indications	cholecystitis, gallstones, biliary ascariasis, migraine, herpes zoster, otitis media, tinnitus, hearing loss, acute pancreatitis.

3. Kidney

Position	inferior to the origin of the superior and inferior crus of the antihelix.
Indications	lumbago, tinnitus, neurasthenia, pyelitis, asthma, nocturnal enureisis, irregular menstruation, nocturnal emission, premature ejaculation.

4. Bladder

Position	on the anterior inferior of the inferior crus of the antihelix.
Indications	cystitis, enuresis, urinary retention, lumbago, sciatica, post-headache.

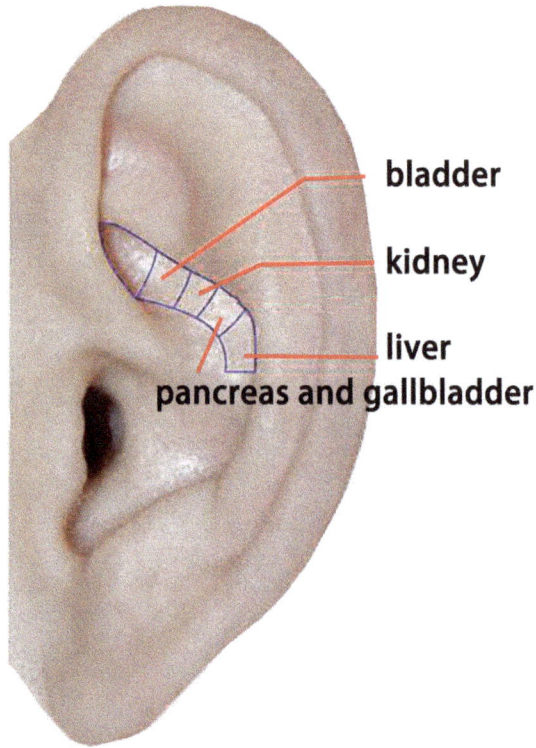

Figure 3-15 liver—bladder

5. Ureter

Position	between Kidney and Bladder.
Indications	ureterolal colic.

6. Angle of superior concha

Position	on the posterior superior angle of the cymba concha.
Indications	prostatitis, urethritis.

7. Center of superior concha

Position	on the center of the cymba concha.
Indications	abdominal pain, bloating, biliary ascariasis, parotitis.

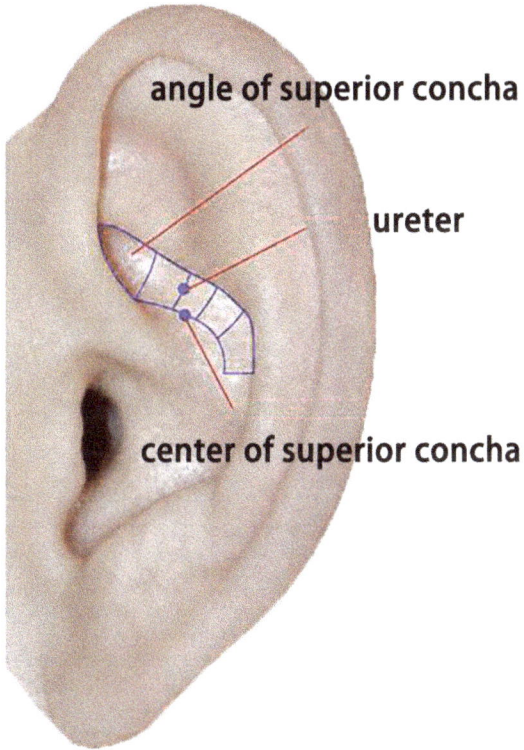

Figure 3-16 ureter—center of superior concha

Part XII Eight points on the ear lobe

The frontal surface of the lobe is divided by three equidistant vertical lines extending from the lower border of the cartilage of the notch between the tragus and the antitragus to the lower lobe, and placing two equidistant horizontal lines on the 2nd vertical line to divide the lobe into nine areas from top to bottom and from front to back.

1. Tooth

Position	on the first part of the ear lobe.
Indications	toothache, periodontitis, hypotension.

2. Tongue

Position	on the second part of the ear lobe.
Indications	glossitis, stomatitis.

3. Jaw

Position	on the third part of the ear lobe.
Indications	toothache, dysfunction of the temporomandibular joint.

4. Anterior ear lobe

Position	on the fourth part of the ear lobe.
Indications	neurosism, toothache.

5. Eye

Position	on the fifth part of the ear lobe.
Indications	acute conjunctivitis, electric opthaimia, stye, pseudo-myopia.

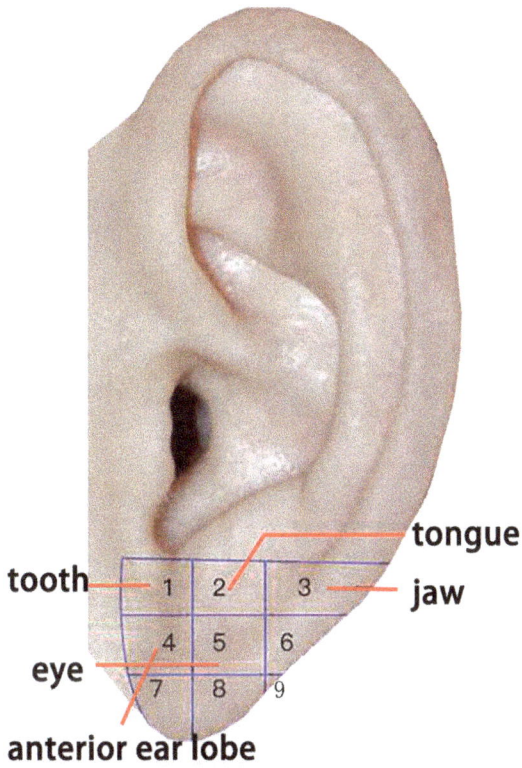

Figure 3-17 tooth—eye

6. Internal ear

Position	on the sixth part of the ear lobe.
Indications	Meniere's disease, tinnitus, hearing loss.

7. Cheek

Position	it is located surrounding at the juncture of LO5 and LO6.
Indications	peripheral facial paralysis, trigeminal neuralgia, acne, flat warts.

8. Tonsil

Position	on the seventh, eighth and ninth part of the ear lobe.
Indications	Tonsillitis, pharyngitis.

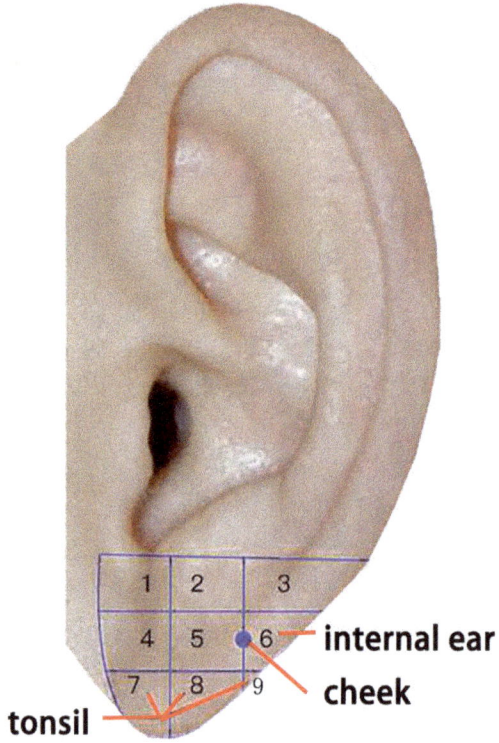

Figure 3-18 internal ear—tonsil

Quarte XIII Nine points on the posteromedial surface of the ear

1. Upper ear root

Position	on the highest part of the ear root.
Indications	epistaxis.

2. Root of ear vagus

Position	on the juncture of the posteromedial surface of the ear and the mastoid process, corresponding to the crus of the helix.
Indications	cholecystitis, gallstones, biliary ascariasis, nasal congestion, tachycardia, abdominal pain, diarrhea.

3. Lower ear root

Position	on the lowest part of the ear root.
Indications	hypotension.

4. Groove, posteromedial surface

Position	The groove in the shape of "Y" on the posteromedial surface of the ear formed by the superior and inferior crura of the antihelix and the body of the antihelix.
Indications	hypertension, cutaneous pruritus.

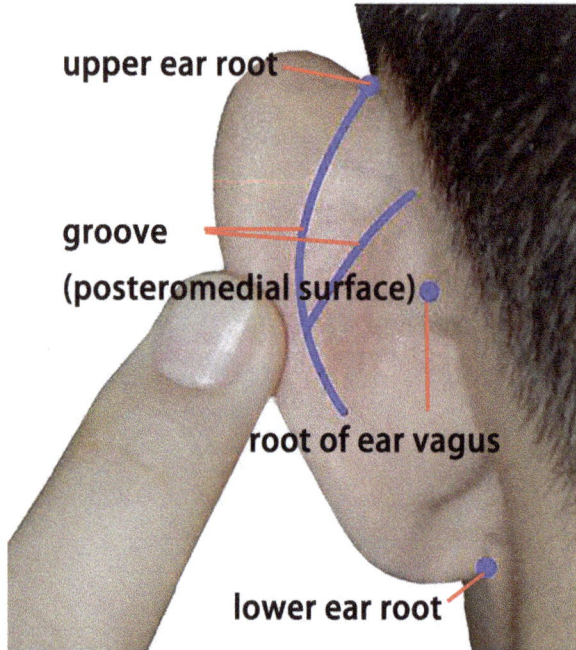

Figure 3-19 upper ear root— groove, posteromedial surface

5. Heart, posteromedial surface

Position	on the upper part of the posteromedial surface of the ear.
Indications	heart palpitations, insomnia, nightmares.

6. Spleen, posteromedial surface

Position	on the posteromedial surface of the ear close to the terminus of the helix crus.
Indications	stomach pain, indigestion, poor appetite.

7. Liver, posteromedial surface

Position	on the posteromedial surface of the auricle lateral to Spleen of posteromedial Surface.
Indications	cholecystitis, gallstones, hypochondriac pain.

8. Lung, posteromedial surface

Position	on the posteromedial surface of the auricle medial to spleen of posteromedial Surface.
Indications	cough, pruritus.

9. Kidney, posteromedial surface

Position	on the inferior part of the posteromedial surface of the ear.
Indications	headache, dizziness, neurasthenia.

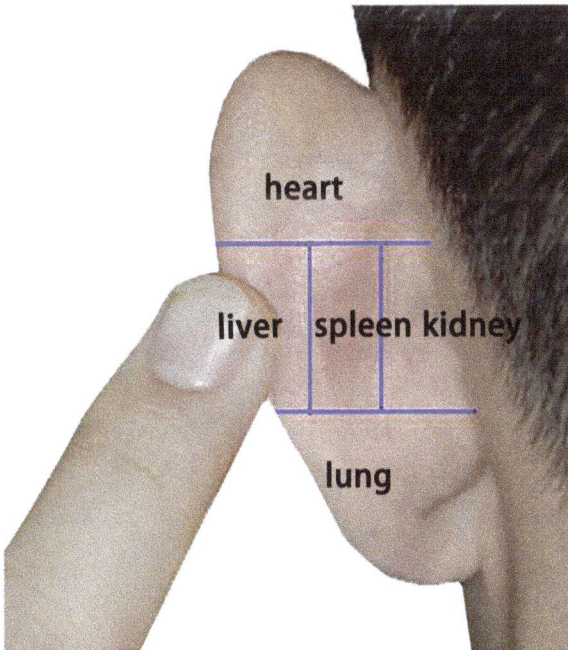

Figure 3-20 heart, posteromedial surface—kidney, posteromedial surface

Reflex zones of the hands

Reflex zones of the hands therapy is a method to treat diseases by stimulating the reflex zones of the hands.

1. Frontal sinus

Position	at the fire fingertips of the palm.
Indications	the stroke, concussion, sinusitis, dizziness, headache, colds, fever, insomnia, eyes, ears, nose and mouth diseases.

2. Brain (head)

Position	At the thumb pulp of the palm.
Indications	concussion, stroke, cerebral palsy, cerebral thrombosis, dizziness, headache, cold, confusion, neurasthenia, respiratory, visual impairment.

3. Pituitary

Position	in the center of thumb pulp.
Indications	dysfunction of the thyroid, parathyroid, adrenal gland, gonads, spleen, pancreas, etc., children stunted, menopausal syndrome.

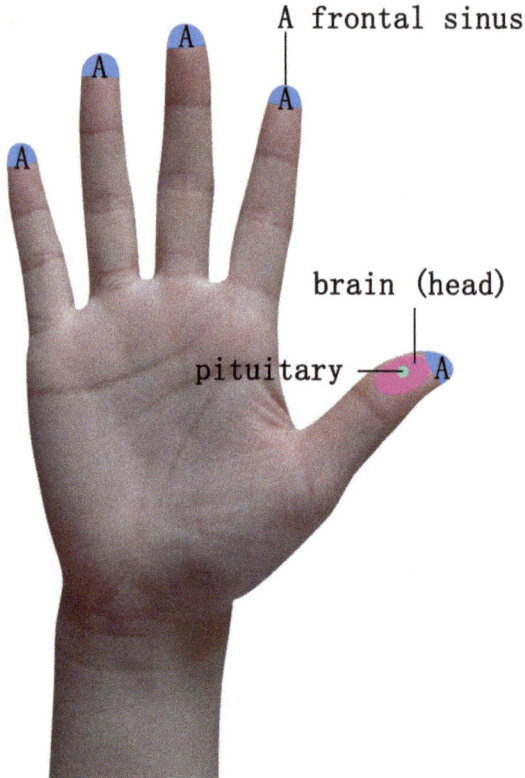

A frontal sinus

A

A

A

A

A

brain (head)

pituitary — A

Figure 4-1 frontal sinus—pituitary

4. Nose

Position	at the junction of the red and white skin of the radial side of the thumb section II.
Indications	nasal congestion, runny nose, epistaxis (bleeding contraindications), sinusitis, allergic rhinitis, acute and chronic rhinitis and upper respiratory tract infection.

5. Tonsil

Position	on both sides of the hands, the dorsal tendon of the thumb section II.
Indications	tonsillitis, upper respiratory tract infection, fever.

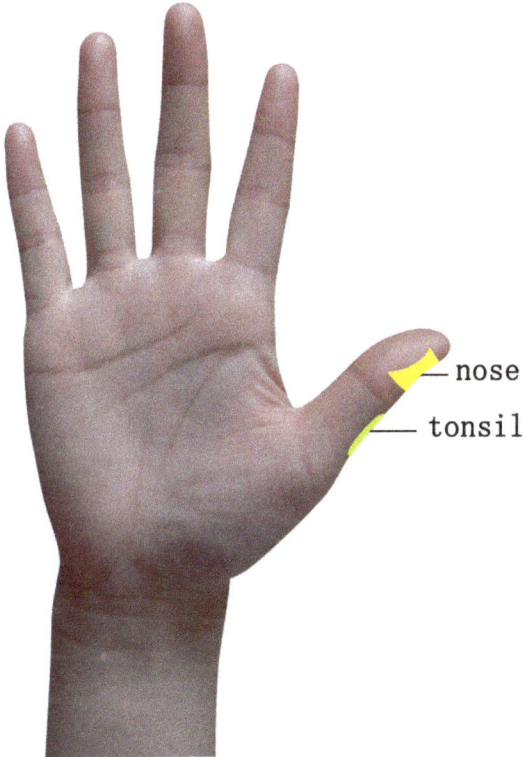

Figure 4-2 nose— tonsil

6. Esophagus, trachea

Position	at the radial side of the thumb section II of hands, at the junction of the red and white skin.
Indications	esophagitis, esophageal cancer, bronchitis

7. Chest respiratory area

Position	in the palm of hands, the area between the crease of thumb interphalangeal joint and the crease of wrist.
Indications	chest tightness, wheezing, cough, pneumonia, bronchitis, asthma.

8. Stomach

Position	located at the far-end of the first metacarpal bone of hands.
Indications	stomach pain, bloating, hyperacidity, indigestion, ptosis of the stomach, nausea, vomiting, acute and chronic gastritis.

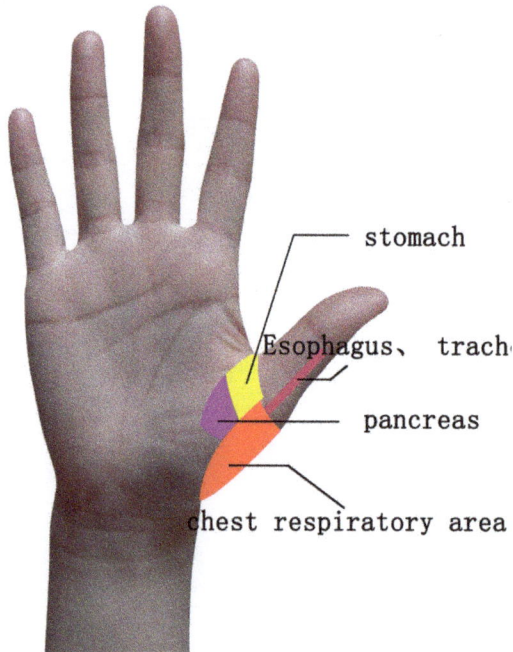

Figure 4-3 Esophagus—pancreas

9. Pancreas

Position	located between reflex zones of the stomach and reflex zones of duodenum, the middle part of the first meta-carpal bone.
Indications	pancreatitis, diabetes, indigestion.

10. Duodenum

Position	located in the palm, near-end of the first metacarpal bone, under the reflex zones of pancreas.
Indications	duodenal ulcers, loss of appetite, indigestion, bloating, food poisoning.

11. Thyroid

Position	located in the palm, between the first and second meta-carpal bone, from nearly heart end to the direction of the first web, showing as a curved belt area.
Indications	hyperthyroidism or lower, thyroiditis, heart palpitations, insomnia, colds, irritability, and obesity.

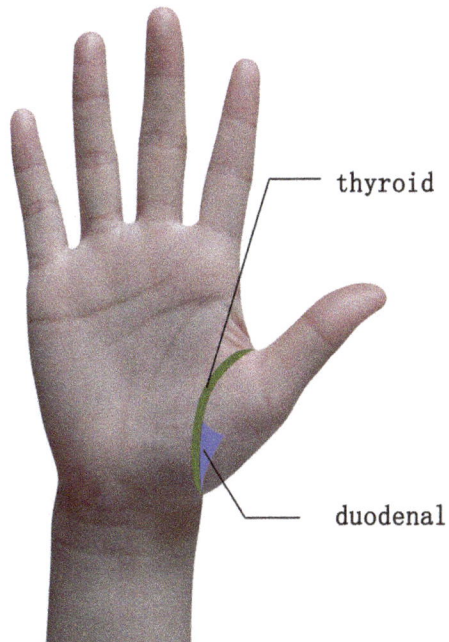

Figure 4-4 duodenal—thyroid

12. Eye

Position	at the roots of fingers between the second and the third finger of palm and back of hands.
Indications	conjunctivitis, keratitis, myopia, hyperopia, glaucoma, cataracts, photophobia, tearing, presbyopia, retinal hemorrhage.

13. Ear

Position	at roots of fingers between the fourth and the fifth finger of palm and back of hands.
Indications	tinnitus, otitis media, hearing loss.

14. Trapezius

Position	in the cross-belt area, under the reflex zones of eye and ear, at the side of palm.
Indications	neck, shoulder, back pain, cervical spondylosis, stiff neck.

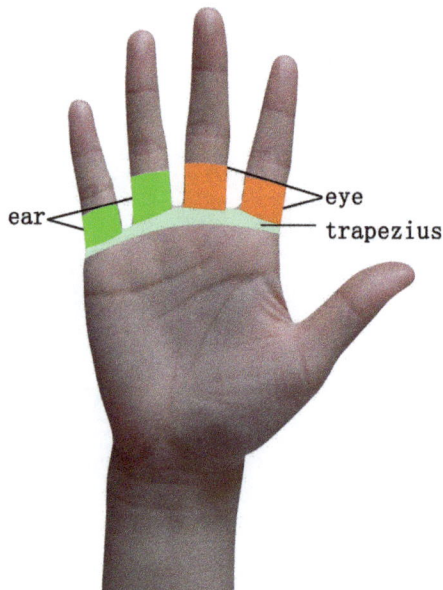

Figure 4-5 eye—trapezius

15. Neck and shoulder District

Position	at both sides of near-end finger bone of roots of fingers of hands and the connection parts of the metacarpophalangeal joints. The back of the hand represents the back bone of neck and shoulder. The palm of hand is before zone of neck and shoulder.
Indications	the shoulder and neck pain, such as frozen shoulder, cervical spondylosis, shoulder and neck fasciitis, stiff neck.

16. Neck

Position	at the side of palm and back of near-end of thumb of hands.
Indications	neck pain, stiff neck, dizziness, headache, nosebleeds, hypertension, stiff neck.

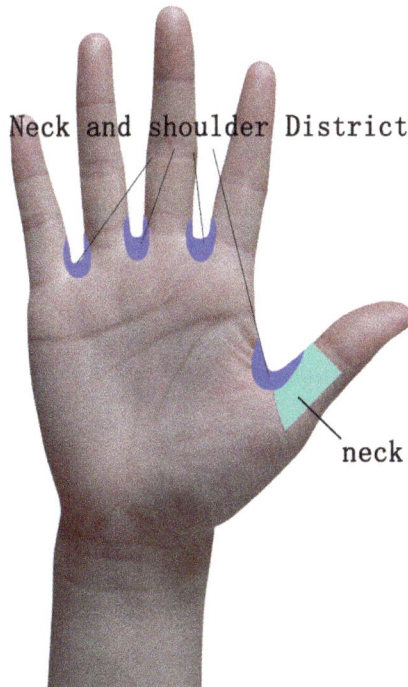

Neck and shoulder District

neck

Figure 4-6 Neck and shoulder District—neck

17. Bladder

Position	located in the hollow of the occasion of big and small thenars in the palm.
Indications	cystitis, urethritis, bladder stones, hypertension, atherosclerosis, urinary system and other bladder disorders.

18. Ureter

Position	located in the belt area between reflex zones of the bladder and reflex zone of the kidney in the palm.
Indications	ureteritis, ureteral calculi, ureteral stenosis, hypertension, arteriosclerosis, rheumatism, urinary system infection.

19. Kidney

Position	located at the midpoint of the third metacarpal bone in the palm, that is, the palm of the hand, at the equivalent of the location of laogong point (PC 8).
Indications	nephritis, kidney stones, wandering kidney, renal insufficiency, uremia, low back pain, urinary tract infections, hypertension, edema.

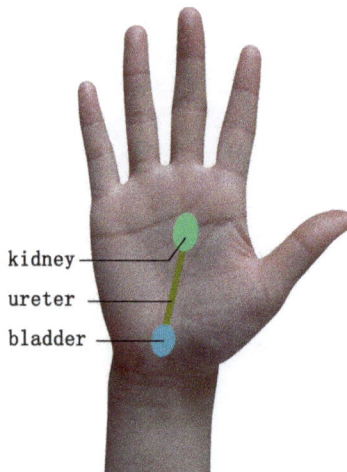

kidney
ureter
bladder

Figure 4-7 bladder—kidney

20. Adrenal

Position	located on the side of the palm of pairs of hands, the far-end between the second and third metacarpal bone.
Indications	dizziness, high blood pressure, the tip of finger paralysis, palms sweating, hands hot, adrenal cortex imperfecta.

21. Celiac plexus

Position	located on the side of the palm of pairs of hands, among the metacarpal bone of the second, third and fourth, on both sides of reflex zones of kidney.
Indications	gastrointestinal disorders, abdominal pain, bloating, diarrhea, hiccups, menopausal syndrome, irritability, insomnia and so on.

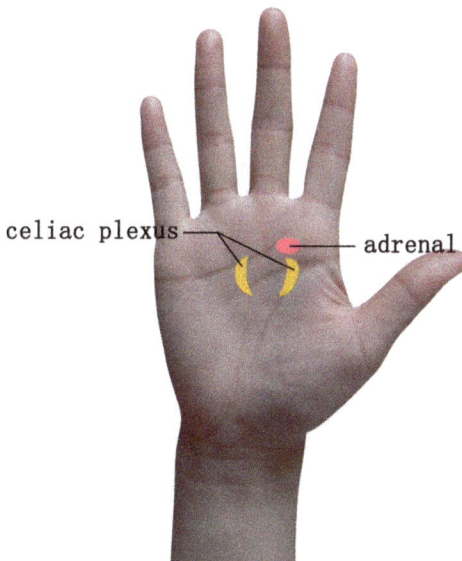

Figure 4-8 adrenal—celiac plexus

22. Ascending colon

Position	on the side of palm of hand, the belt area which parallels to the level of the first web, that is arrived by the part between the fourth and the fifth metacarpal bone.
Indications	constipation, abdominal pain, colitis, diarrhea.

24. Transverse colon

Position	it is located on the side of palm of right hand, the belt area between the up-end of reflex zone of the ascending colon and first web; on the side of palm of left hand, the belt area between first web and the descending colon.
Indications	diarrhea, abdominal distention, abdominal pain, colitis, constipation.

25. Small intestine

Position	located in the hollow of the center of palm of pairs hands, the part surrounded by reflex zones of colons.
Indications	acute and chronic enteritis, indigestion, loss of appetite, stomach bulge nausea.

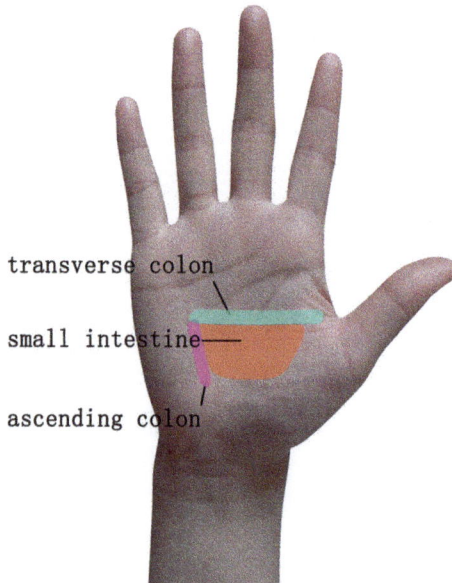

Figure 4-9 Ascending colon—small intestine

25. Ileocecal valve

Position	located on the side of palm of right hand, the radial side of connection part between the bottom of the fourth and fifth metacarpal bone and hamate bone.
Indications	abdominal distension, abdominal pain.

26. Cecum, appendix

Position	located on the side of palm of right hand, the ulnar side of connection part between the bottom of the fourth and fifth metacarpal bone and hamate bone.
Indications	bloating, diarrhea, indigestion, appendicitis.

27. Stomach, spleen, large intestine area

Position	located in the palms of pairs of hands, the oval-shaped area between the first and second metacarpal bone.
Indications	indigestion, loss of appetite, abdominal pain, bloating, diarrhea, enteritis, constipation.

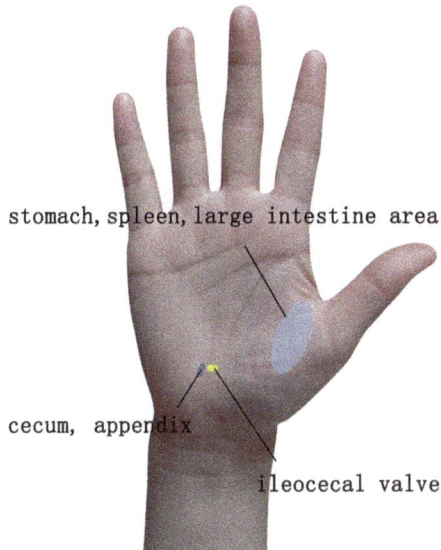

stomach, spleen, large intestine area

cecum, appendix

ileocecal valve

Figure 4-10 ileocecal valve—stomach, spleen, large intestine area

28. Lung, bronchus

Position	reflex zones of lung is located in the palm, across the second, third, fourth, fifth metacarpal bone, the belt area near the metacarpophalangeal joint; reflex zones of bronchus is located in the third section of middle finger bone.
Indications	pneumonia, bronchitis, emphysema, tuberculosis, lung cancer, chest tightness.

29. Liver

Position	located on the side of palm of right hand, the tip of the metacarpal bone between the fourth and the fifth metacarpal bone.
Indications	hepatitis, cirrhosis, abdominal pain, indigestion, bloating, dizziness, eye, etc.

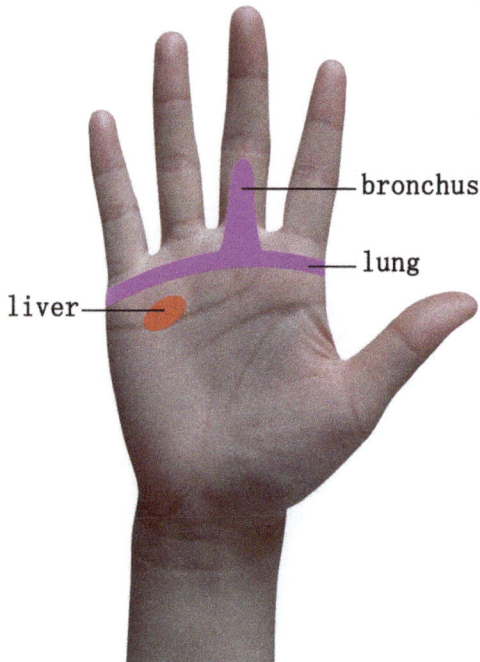

Figure 4-11 lung—liver

30. Gallbladder

Position	located on the side of palm of right hand, between the fourth and fifth metacarpal bones, the bottom of the wrist side reflex zones of the liver.
Indications	Cholecystitis, cholelithiasis, bile duct ascariasis, anorexia, dyspepsia, gastrointestinal disorders, hyperlipidemia, and acne.

31. Gonads (ovaries, testicles)

Position	located at the root of the pairs of hands, the middle of the wrist crease, equivalent to daling point (PC 7).
Indications	sexual dysfunction, infertility, benign prostatic hyperplasia, irregular menstruation, dysmenorrhea.

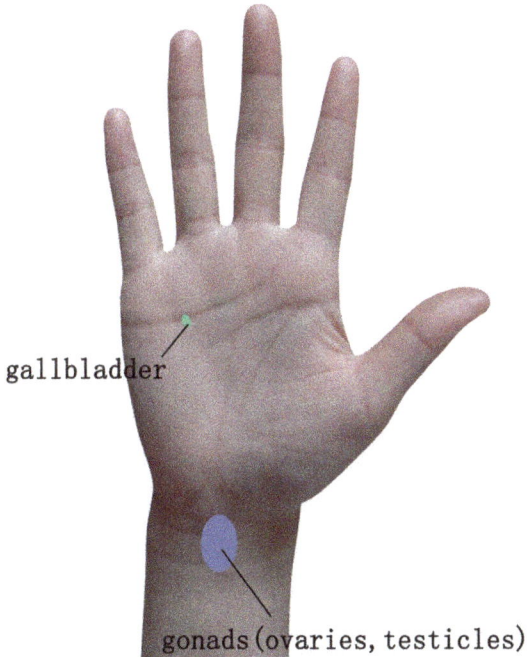

gallbladder

gonads (ovaries, testicles)

Figure 4-12 gallbladder—gonads (ovaries, testicles)

32. Prostate, uterus, vagina, urethra

Position	located on the wrist crease of pairs of hands, the belt area of both sides of reflex zones of gonads.
Indications	benign prostatic hyperplasia, prostatitis, uterine fibroids, endometritis, cervicitis, vaginitis, abnormal vaginal discharge, urethritis, urinary tract infections, etc.

33. Groin

Position	located at the radial side of the wrist crease of palm side of pairs of hands, in the depression of the radial head. Equivalent of taiyuan point (LU 9).
Indications	sexual dysfunction, benign prostatic hyperplasia, reproductive system disease, hernia, abdominal pain.

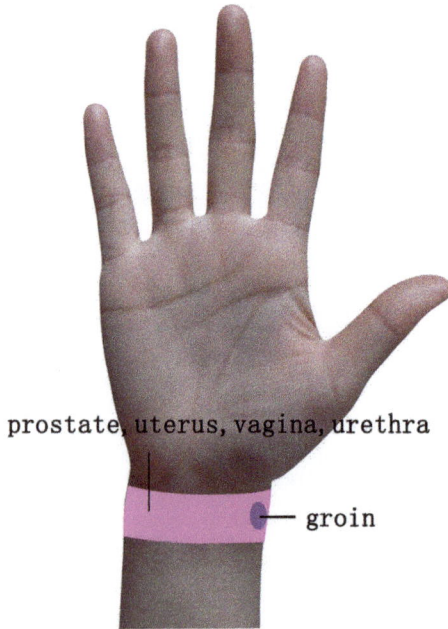

prostate, uterus, vagina, urethra

groin

Figure 4-13 prostate—groin

34. Heart

Position	located at the ulnar side of left hand, between the fourth and fifth metacarpal bone of palm and back of hand, the distal place of metacarpal bone.
Indications	arrhythmia, angina, palpitations, chest tightness, high blood pressure, low blood pressure, heart defects and diseases of the circulatory system.

35. Spleen

Position	located at the palm of left hand, the remote place between the fourth and fifth metacarpal bone.
Indications	loss of appetite, indigestion, fever, inflammation, and anemia.

36. Descending colon

Position	located at the palm of left hand, between the fourth, fifth metacarpal bone, the belt area between the first web and the hamate bone.
Indications	diarrhea, abdominal pain, bloating, colitis, constipation.

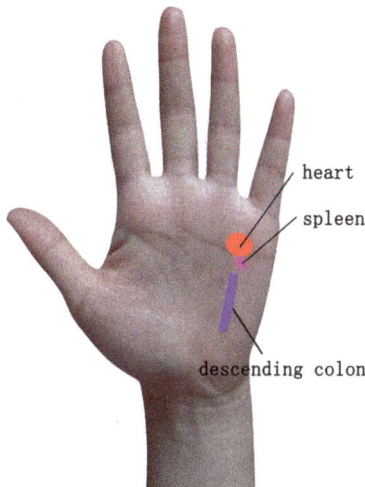

Figure 4-14 heart—descending colon

37. Sigmoid colon

Position	located at the palm of left hand, the belt area between the carpometacarpal joints, which is the connection of the end of fifth metacarpal bone and hamate bone and the connection of the first and second metacarpal bone.
Indications	abdominal pain, bloating, diarrhea, enteritis, constipation.

38. Anal canal, anal

Position	located at the palm of left hand, at the second carpometacarpal joint, that is, the end of the reflex zones of sigmoid.
Indications	constipation, rectal prolapse, hemorrhoids.

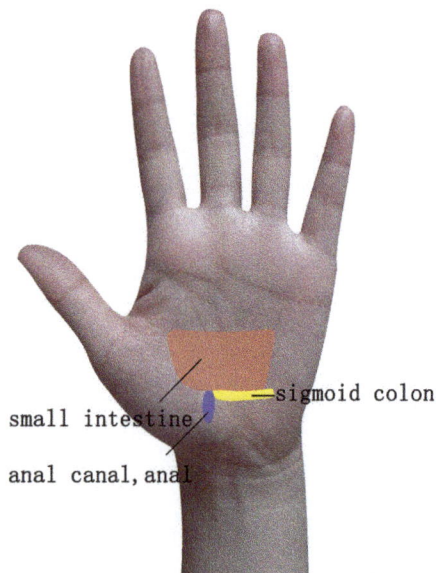

small intestine

sigmoid colon

anal canal, anal

Figure 4-15 sigmoid colon—anal

39. Cerebellum, brainstem

Position	located in the palm, ulnar side of thumb palm.
Indications	concussion, high blood pressure, dizziness, headache, insomnia, cold, shaking walking, muscle tension, tendon and joint diseases.

40. The trigeminal nerve

Position	located in the palm, the remote end of the ulnar edge of thumb pulp, the upright of reflex zones of cerebellum and brainstem.
Indications	the facial nerve paralysis, migraine, head weight, insomnia, flu, mumps, eyes, ears, mouth caused by neuralgia.

41. Maxillary and mandibular

Position	located at the back of thumb pairs of hands, the belt region of the up and down of crease of thumb interphalangeal joint. The distal is higher jaw, the proximal is lower jaw.
Indications	temporomandibular joint disorders, periodontitis, gingivitis, tooth decay, oral ulcers.

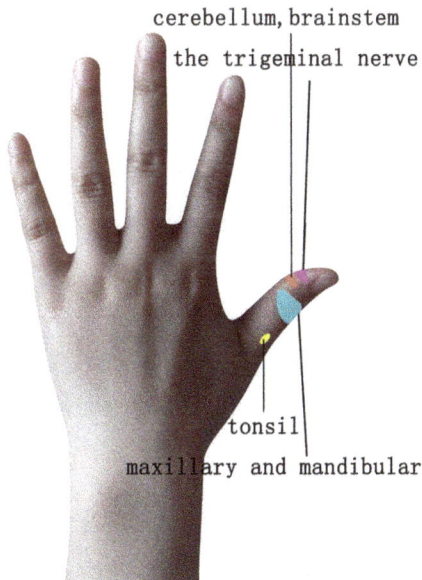

cerebellum, brainstem
the trigeminal nerve
tonsil
maxillary and mandibular

Figure 4-16 cerebellum—maxillary and mandibular

42. Tongue

Position	located on the back of thumb of pairs of hands, the Center of crease of interphalangeal joint.
Indications	oral ulcers, dysgeusia.

43. Larynx, trachea

Position	located in the center of the back of the proximal phalanx of thumbs of pairs of hands.
Indications	the upper respiratory tract infections, laryngitis, bronchitis, cough, shortness of breath.

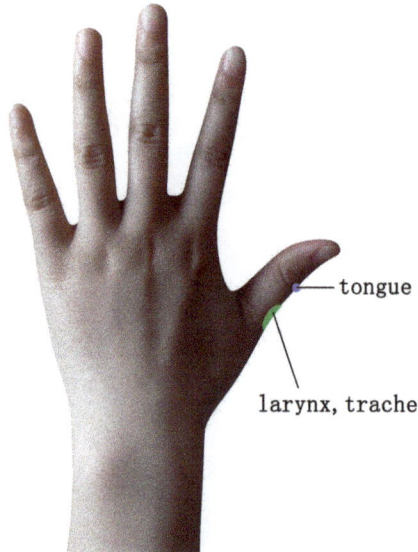

Figure 4-17 tongue—trachea

44. Spine

Position	located at the body of the first, second, third, fourth and fifth metacarpal bone of the back of hand.
Indications	cervical spondylosis, stiff neck, back pain, low back pain.

45. Cervical

Position	located at the back of hand, the distal 1/5 of the back side of metacarpal bones of all.
Indications	neck stiffness, neck pain, dizziness, headache, stiff neck, a variety of cervical lesions.

46. Thoracic

Position	located at the back of hand, the middle 2/5 of the back side of metacarpal bones of all.
Indications	the shoulder pain, thoracic bone spurs, lumbar pain, thoracic disc herniation, chest tightness, chest pain.

47. Lumbar

Position	located at the back of hand, the proximal 2/5 of the back side of metacarpal bones of all.
Indications	back pain, lumbar spine bone spurs, lumbar pain, lumbar tip disc hernia, lumbar muscle strain.

A:cervical B:thoracic C:lumbar

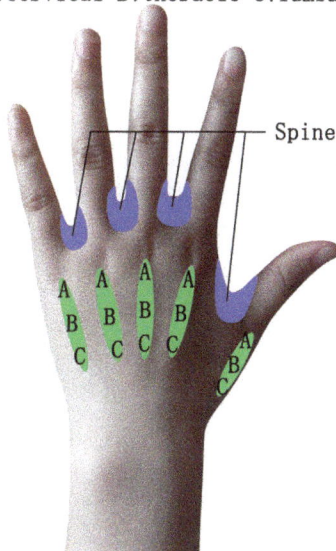

Figure 4-18 spine—lumbar

48. Sacrum

Position	located at the back of hand, the connections of carpo-metacarpal joints of all.
Indications	the sacrum injury, sacrum bone spurs, sciatica.

49. Coccyx

Position	located at the back of hand, the crease of back of wrist.
Indications	sciatica, tailbone injury sequelae.

50. Ribs

Position	located at the back of pairs of hands, the inner reflex zones of ribs is located at the radial side of the middle of the remote edge of the body of the second metacarpal bone; the outer reflex zone of ribs is located between the fourth and fifth metacarpal bone, the hollow near the end of the metacarpal bone.
Indications	pleurisy, chest tightness, pleurisy, rib injury.

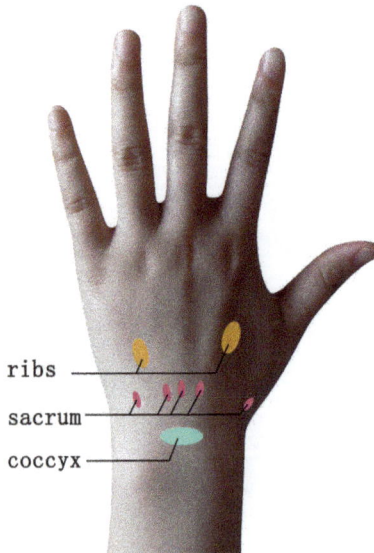

Figure 4-19 sacrum—ribs

51. The labyrinth

Position	located at the back of pairs of hands, among the third, fourth, fifth metacarpophalangeal joints, the connection among the third, fourth, fifth finger roots.
Indications	dizziness, tinnitus, Meniere's syndrome, motion sickness, high blood pressure, low blood pressure, balance disorders.

52. Chest, breast

Position	located at the back of hands, the remote edge of the second, third and fourth metacarpal bone.
Indications	chest diseases, respiratory diseases, heart disease, breast disease.

54. Diaphragm

Position	located at the back of pairs of hands, the belt region across the middle of the second, third and fourth metacarpal bone.
Indications	hiccups, nausea, vomiting, abdominal distention, abdominal pain.

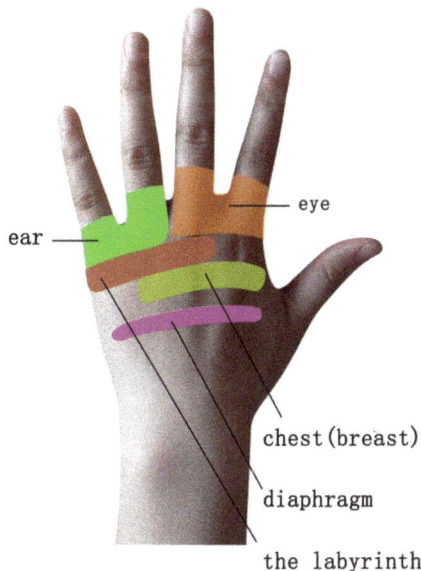

Figure 4-20 the labyrinth—diaphragm

54. Blood pressure district

Position	located at the back of the hand, the enclosed region between the first and second metacarpal bone and yangxi point (LI 5), and the radial side of the proximal phalanx of inner finger.
Indications	hypertension, hypotension, dizziness, headache.

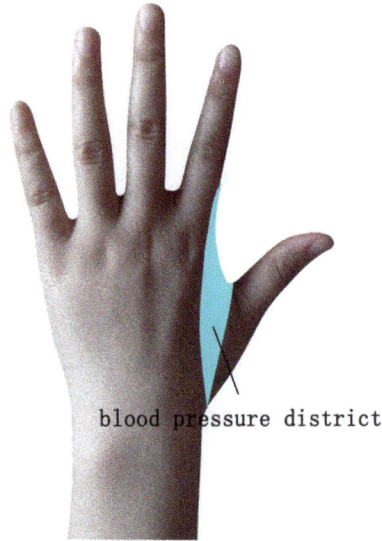

blood pressure district

Figure 4-21 blood pressure district

55. Shoulder

Position	located at the junction of the red and white skin after the metacarpophalangeal joint of the little finger.
Indications	frozen shoulder, arm pain, numbness in the hands of cataract.

56. Elbow

Position	located at the back of hand, the ulnar side of the center of the body, the fifth metacarpal bone.
Indications	the elbow disease (such as tennis elbow, olecranon bursitis, medial epicondyle), upper limb paralysis, arm numbness.

57. Knee

Position	located in the hollow between the proximal ulnar edge of the fifth metacarpal bone and the carpal.
Indications	the knee lesions, lower limb paralysis.

58. Hip

Position	located at the back of hand, around the surface of ulnar and radial styloid bone.
Indications	the hip joint disease, sciatica, low back pain.

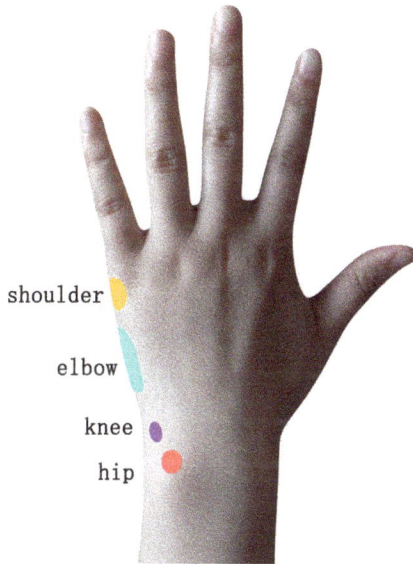

Figure 4-22 shoulder—hip

59. Head and neck lymph nodes

Position	located in the hollow of the palm and back side of all of finger roots of pairs of hands.
Indications	cervical lymph node enlargement, goiter, hyperthyroidism, and toothache.

60. Parathyroid

Position	located in the hollow of back side of the first metacarpophalangeal joint of the radial side of pairs of hands.
Indications	allergies, cramps, insomnia, vomiting, nausea, hypocalcemia, brittle nails, seizures.

61. Thymus lymph nodes

Position	located at the ulnar edge of the first metacarpophalangeal joint.
Indications	fever, inflammation, cysts, strengthen the immune cancer-fighting ability.

62. Upper body lymph nodes

Position	located at the back of the hand, the junction of the lunate, triquetrum and ulna.
Indications	fever, inflammation, and cysts. May enhance the immune anti-cancer ability.

Figure 4-23 head and neck lymph nodes—upper body lymph nodes

63. Lower body lymph nodes

Position	located at the back of hand, the junction of the scaphoid and the radius.
Indications	fever, inflammation, and cysts.

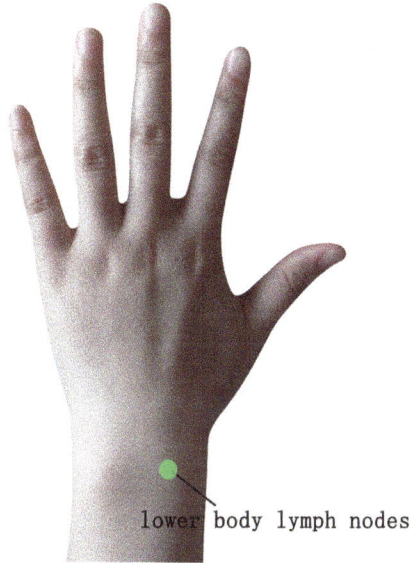

lower body lymph nodes

Figure 4-24 lower body lymph nodes

CHAPTER 𝔜

Reflex zones of the feet

Reflex zone of foot therapy is to treat diseases by stimulating the reflex zones on feet.

1. Brain

Position	located at all of hallux pulp of each feet. Left encephalopathy massage right foot; right encephalopathy massage left foot.
Indications	concussion, stroke, cerebral palsy, cerebral thrombosis, dizziness, headache, cold, confusion, neurasthenia, visual impairment

2. Nose

Position	reflex zone of nose is located out of the hallux pulp of pair of feet, near the upright of the hallux till the roots, the left nose disease massage right foot; the right nose disease massage left foot.
Indications	nasal congestion, runny nose, epistaxis (bleeding contra indications), sinusitis, allergic rhinitis, acute and chronic rhinitis and upper respiratory tract infection.

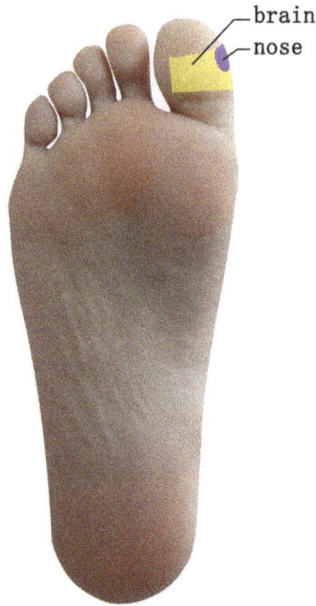

Figure 5-1 brain—nose

3. Frontal sinus

Position	located at the pulp of ten toes.
Indications	the stroke, concussion, sinusitis, dizziness, headache, colds, fever, insomnia, eyes, ears, nose and mouth disease.

4. Cerebellum, brainstem,

Position	reflex zones of cerebellar is located at the right side of foot of root of section I of the big toe, near the second toe.
Indications	concussion, high blood pressure, dizziness, headache, insomnia, cold, shaking walking, muscle tension, tendon and joint diseases.

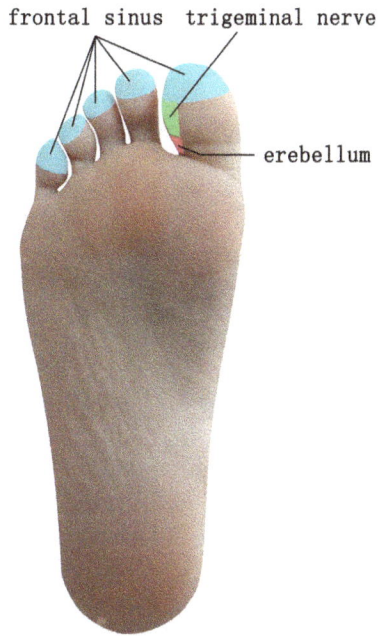

Figure 5-2 frontal sinus—trigeminal nerve

5. Trigeminal nerve

Position	located at the outer of hallux of pair of feet, near the second toe.
Indications	the facial nerve paralysis, migraine, head weight, insomnia, flu, mumps, eyes, ears, mouth caused by neuralgia.

6. Pituitary

Position	located in the center of hallux pulp of pair of feet.
Indications	dysfunction of the thyroid, parathyroid, adrenal gland, gonads, spleen, pancreas, etc., children stunted, menopausal syndrome.

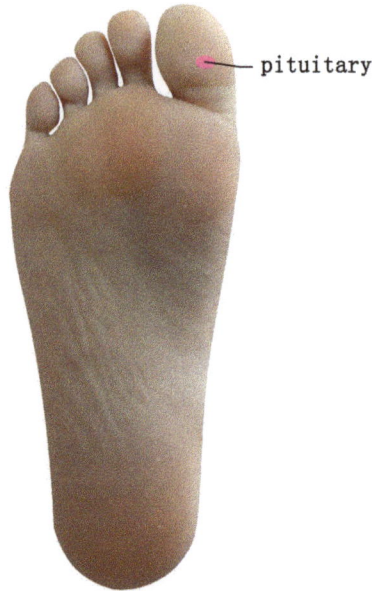

pituitary

Figure 5-3 pituitary

7. Eye

Position	at the middle and proximal section of the second and third toe of pair of feet; left eye disease massage right foot, right eye disease massage left foot.
Indications	conjunctivitis, keratitis, myopia, hyperopia, glaucoma, cataracts, photophobia, lacrimation, presbyopia, retinal hemorrhage.

8. Ear

Position	located at the middle and proximal section of the fourth and fifth toe of pair of feet. Left ear disease massage right foot. Right ear disease massage left foot.
Indications	tinnitus, otitis media, hearing loss.

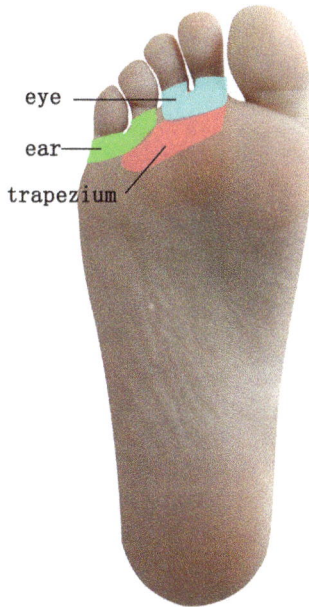

Figure 5-4 eye—trapeziums

9. Trapeziums

Position	below the second, three and fourth metatarso-phalangeal joints of palm of feet, as a horizontal ribbon.
Indications	frozen shoulder, shoulder pain, arms weakness, numbness in the hand, stiff neck, eye cataracts.

10. Neck

Position	located at the crease of the bottom of hallux of pair of feet. The left side of neck disease massage the right foot – the right side of neck disease massage left foot.
Indications	neck pain, stiff neck, dizziness, headache, nosebleeds, hypertension, stiff neck.

11. Cervical

Position	located at the end of the crease on the inner phalanx of hallux of both feet.
Indications	neck stiffness, neck pain, dizziness, headache, stiff neck, a variety of cervical lesions.

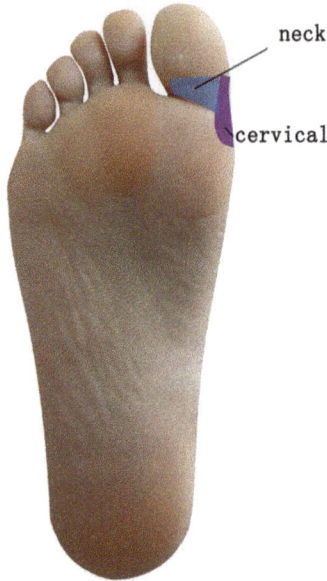

Figure 5-5 neck—cervical

12. Lung and bronchus

Position	similar to the shape of "⊥" area which from the middle part to the middle section of the third toe.
Indications	pneumonia, bronchitis, emphysema, tuberculosis, lung cancer, chest tightness.

13. Adrenal

Position	located slightly outside the top of the second metatarsal of the feet soles.
Indications	inflammation, asthma, allergies, irregular heartbeat, fainting, rheumatism, arthritis, adrenal cortex imperfecta.

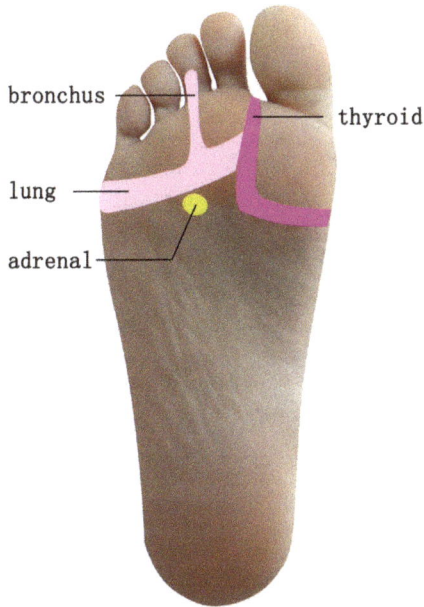

Figure 5-6 lung and bronchus—thyroid

14. Thyroid

Position	similar to the shape of an "L" area, the first half between the first and second metatarsal of the feet soles, which across the middle part of the first metatarsal.
Indications	hyperthyroidism or lower, thyroiditis, heart palpitations, insomnia, colds, irritability, and obesity.

15. Parathyroid

Position	located at the joint of the top of the first metatarsal of the inner edge of the feet soles.
Indications	allergies, cramps, insomnia, vomiting, nausea, hypocalcemia, brittle nails, seizures.

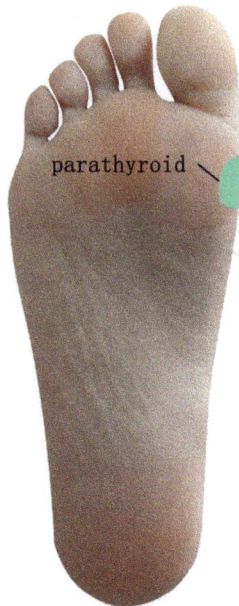

Figure 5-7 parathyroid

16. Esophagus

Position	in the belt region in the joint of the first metatarsophalangeal of the soles of the feet.
Indications	esophagus, esophageal disease.

17. Stomach

Position	located at the middle of the first metatarsal of the feet soles.
Indications	stomach pain, bloating, hyperacidity, indigestion, ptosis of the stomach, nausea, vomiting, acute and chronic gastritis.

18. Pancreas

Position	located at the trailing edge of the first metatarsal body of the feet soles, between the reflex zones of the stomach and duodenum.
Indications	pancreatitis, diabetes, indigestion.

19. Duodenum

Position	located at the place between the bottom of the first metatarsal of the feet soles and the cuneiform joint.
Indications	duodenal ulcers, loss of appetite, indigestion, bloating, food poisoning.

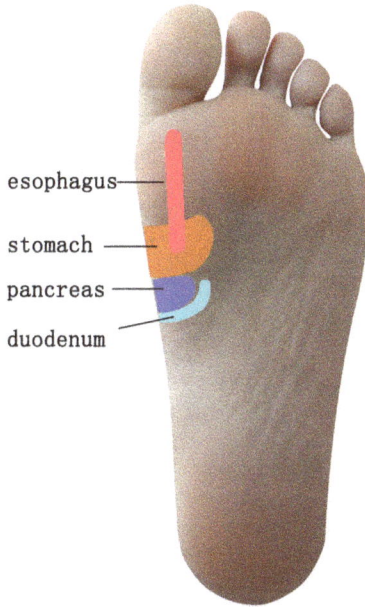

esophagus

stomach

pancreas

duodenum

Figure 5-8 esophagus—duodenum

20. Heart

Position	located on the top of the fourth and fifth metatarsal of the feet soles.
Indications	arrhythmia, angina, palpitations, chest tightness, high blood pressure, low blood pressure, heart defects and diseases of the circulatory system.

21. Spleen

Position	located at the bottom of the fourth and fifth metatarsal of the left foot sole.
Indications	loss of appetite, indigestion, fever, inflammation, and anemia.

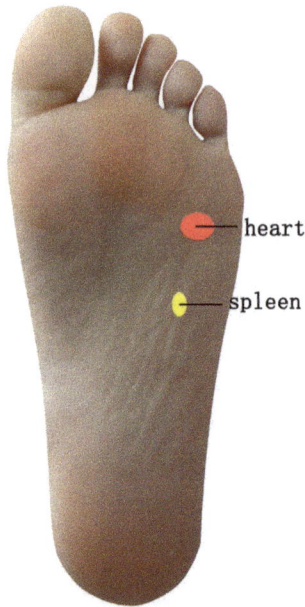

Figure 5-9 heart—spleen

22. Liver

Position	located on the top of the fourth and fifth metatarsal of the right foot sole.
Indications	hepatitis, cirrhosis, hepatomegaly, dry mouth, eye problems, loss of appetite, constipation, gall bladder disease.

23. Gallbladder

Position	located at the middle part of the third and fourth metatarsal of the right foot sole.
Indications	cholecystitis, gallstones, jaundice, liver disease, loss of appetite, constipation.

24. Celiac plexus

Position	located at the middle part of the second, third and fourth metatarsal, which is the center of soles of the feet.
Indications	back pain, chest tightness, hiccups, stomach cramps, bloating.

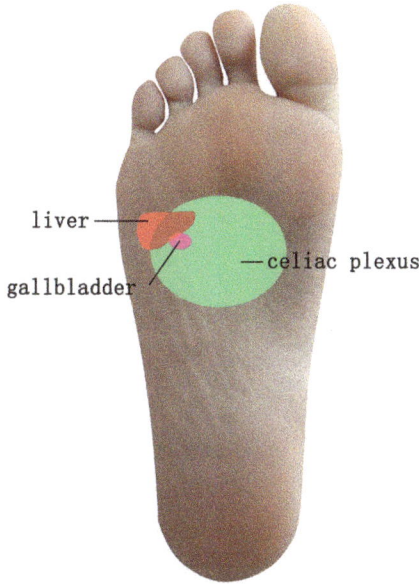

Figure 5-10 liver—celiac plexus

25. Transverse colon

Position	located in the horizontal belt region from the first metatarsal to the bottom of the fifth metatarsal.
Indications	diarrhea, abdominal distention, abdominal pain, colitis, constipation.

26. Ascending colon

Position	located in the belt area out of the reflex zone of the small intestine of the right foot sole.
Indications	constipation, abdominal pain, colitis, diarrhea.

27. Small intestine

Position	located in the central depression of the feet soles, the equivalent part of the cube which is formed by cuneiform, cuboid and navicular.
Indications	acute and chronic enteritis, indigestion, loss of appetite, stomach bulge nausea, abdominal dull pain, fatigue, tension.

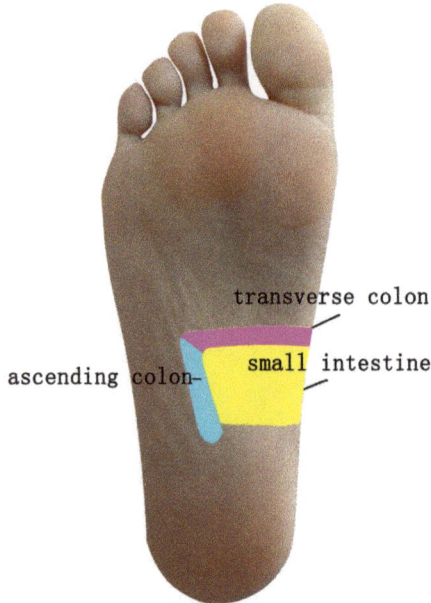

transverse colon

small intestine

ascending colon

Figure 5-11 transverse colon—small intestine

28. Ileocecal valve

Position	located near the outside of the leading edge of calcaneus of the right foot sole, in the front of the reflex zone of cecal appendix.
Indications	digestive system disorders.

29. Cecal appendix

Position	located near the outside of the leading edge of calcaneus of the right foot sole.
Indications	appendicitis, abdominal distension.

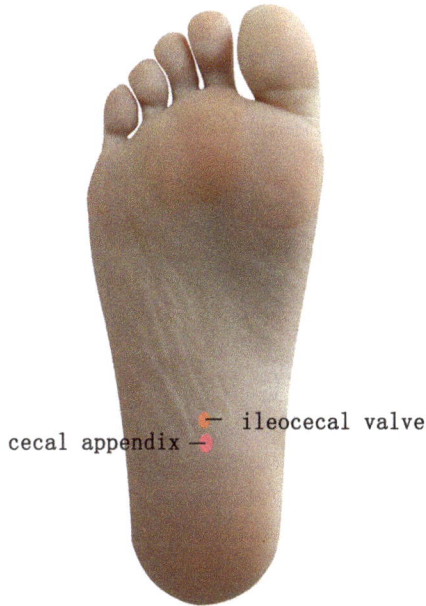

Figure 5-12 ileocecal valve—cecal appendix

30. Descending colon

Position	located in a belt area outside the cuboid of the left foot, sole.
Indications	diarrhea, abdominal pain, bloating, colitis, constipation.

31. Rectum and sigmoid colon

Position	located in a horizontal belt region of the leading edge of the calcaneal of the left foot sole.
Indications	abdominal pain, bloating, diarrhea, enteritis, constipation.

32. Anus

Position	located at the leading edge of the calcaneus of the left foot sole, that is, the end edge of the reflex zones of the rectum and sigmoid colon.
Indications	constipation, rectal prolapse, hemorrhoids.

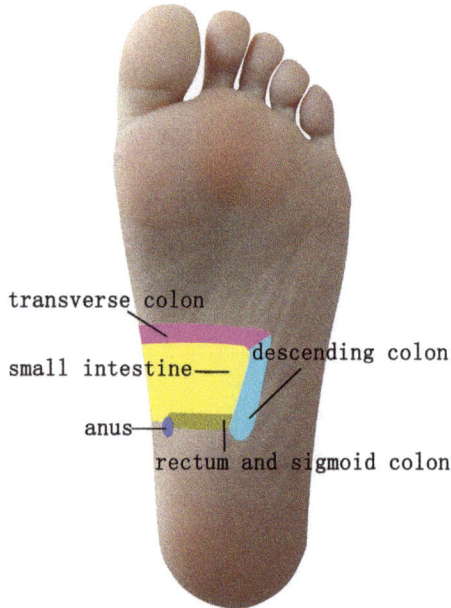

Figure 5-13 descending colon—anus

33. Bladder

Position	located in the front of malleolus medials inside the feet soles, next to the abductor hallucis muscle below the navicular.
Indications	cystitis, urethritis, bladder stones, hypertension, atherosclerosis, urinary system and other bladder disorders.

34. Ureter

Position	located in a region slightly shaped arcuate from the reflex zone of the kidney to the bladder of the feet soles.
Indications	ureteritis, ureteral calculi, ureteral stenosis, hypertension, arteriosclerosis, rheumatism, urinary system infection.

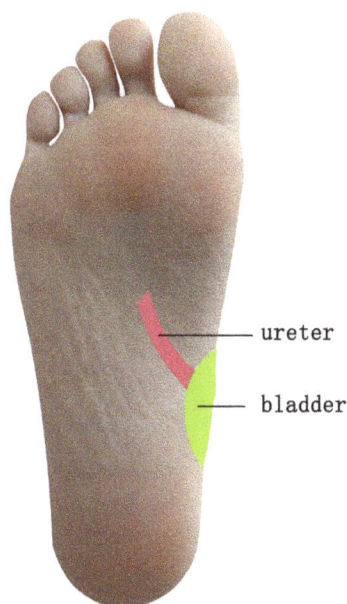

Figure 5-14 bladder—ureter

35. Kidney

Position	located at the joint of the bottom of the second and the third metatarsal of the feet soles.
Indications	nephritis, kidney stones, wandering kidney, renal insufficiency, uremia, low back pain, urinary tract infections, hypertension, edema.

36. Gonads (testes or ovaries)

Position	(1) the center of the heel of the feet soles. (2) In a triangle shaped region below the trailing part of the lateral malleolus of the feet.
Indications	dysmenorrhea, irregular menstruation, infertility, sexual dysfunction, menopause syndrome. Heel central reflex zones can be called "insomnia zone" Insomnia effects.

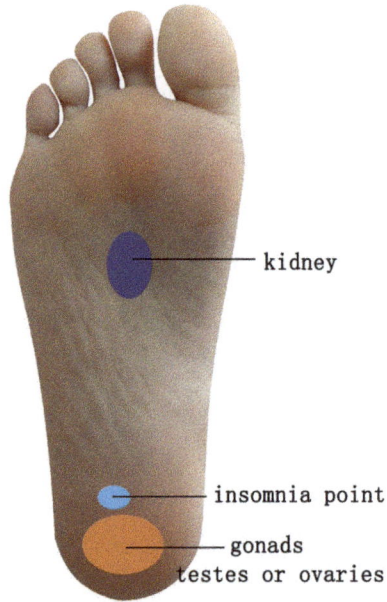

Figure 5-15 kidney—insomnia point

37. Insomnia point

Position	located in the front of the calcaneus at the bottom of the feet, the upright of the reflex zone of gonads. This zone has a better effect for insomnia.
Indications	insomnia, dreams, headache, dizziness.

38. Prostate or uterus

Position	located inside the heel of the feet, a triangle shaped region below the trailing of ankle.
Indications	men: prostatitis, prostatic hypertrophy, urinary frequency, hematuria, dysuria, urethral pain. Women: menstrual pain: irregular menstruation, uterine fibroids, uterine prolapse.

39. Urethra and vagina

Position	located inside the heel of the feet, extended from the reflex zone of the bladder oblique to the place between the talus and navicular.
Indications	urethritis, vaginitis, urinary frequency, enuresis, urinary incontinence, urinary tract infections.

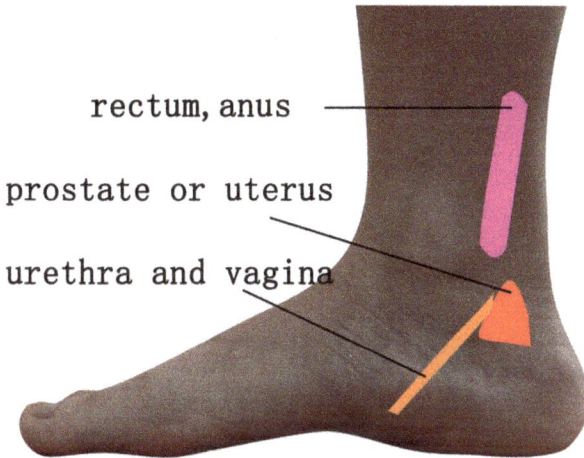

rectum, anus

prostate or uterus

urethra and vagina

Figure 5-16 prostate or uterus—anus

40. Rectum, anus

Position	located in a belt area between the rear of the medial tibial of legs and the flexor digitorum longus tendon, extended from the trailing of lateral malleolus.
Indications	hemorrhoids, proctitis, rectal prolapse, constipation.

41. Groin

Position	located in the depression of the tibial above the ankle angle inside the feet.
Indications	hernia, abdominal pain, reproductive system disorders.

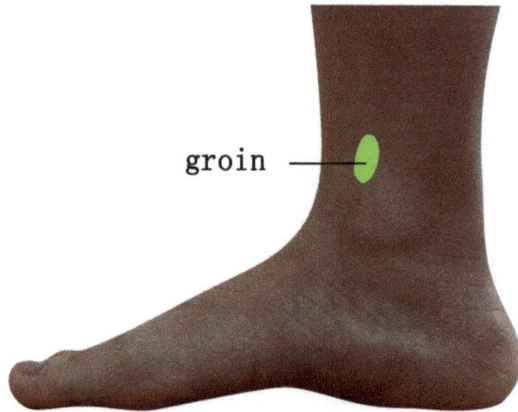

Figure 5-17 groin

42. Sciatic nerve

Position	(1) located from the malleolus medials joint of feet, along the trailing edge of the tibia, extended to pairs of soles upward around. (2) It is located from the lateral malleolus joint of feet, along the front edge of the fibula, extended to the pair of soles, upward around.
Indications	sciatica, sciatic nerve inflammation, foot numbness, foot cramps.

43. Lower abdomen

Position	located at the rear of the fibula outside the feet, the belt region from the rear of lateral malleolus, extending upward about four transverse finger.
Indications	menstrual tension, irregular menstruation, abdominal pain.

44. Diaphragm

Position	located in the front of the cuneiform and cuboid of feet instep, the back-end of the metatarsal, the belt region, which formed by a cross in the instep.
Indications	hiccups, nausea, vomiting, abdominal distention, abdominal pain.

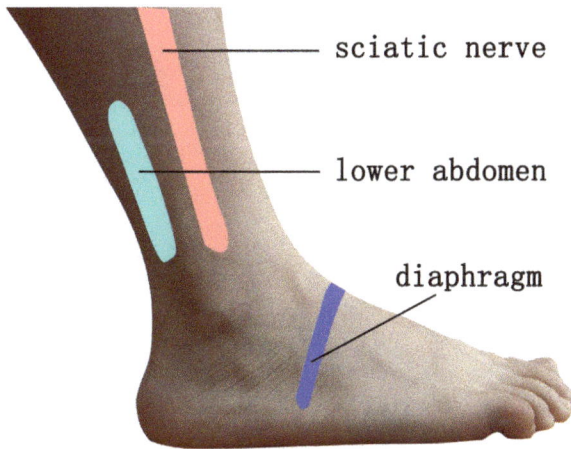

Figure 5-18 sciatic nerve—diaphragm

45. Thoracic

Position	located from the first metatarsal inside feet arches of feet to the cuneiform joint.
Indications	shoulder pain, thoracic bone spurs, lumbar pain, thoracic disc herniation, chest tightness, chest pain.

46. Lumbar

Position	located from the wedge to below edge of the scaphoid inside feet arches of feet.
Indications	back pain, lumbar spine bone spurs, lumbar pain, lumbar tip disc hernia, lumbar muscle strain.

47. Sacrum

Position	located at the following edge of the talus and the calcaneus inside the feet arches of feet.
Indications	sacrum injury, sacrum bone spurs, sciatica.

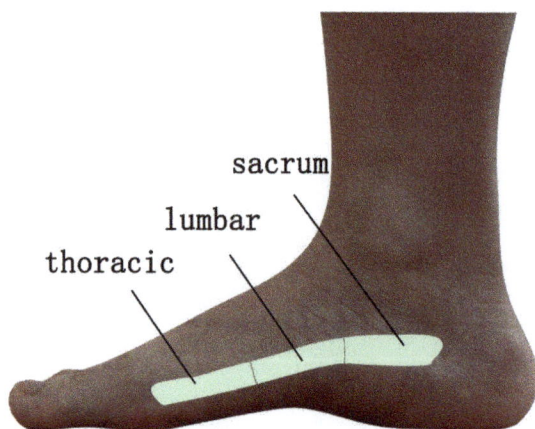

Figure 5-19 thoracic—sacrum

48. Inner coccyx and outer coccyx

Position	located at the tubercle of calcaneal of feet, along the calcaneus from the bottom turning to the top, a region shaped "L", the medial edge is the inner coccyx, the outer edge is the outer coccyx.
Indications	sciatica, tailbone injury sequelae.

49. Hip

Position	located in the four positions, which are located under the malleolus medialis and the lateral malledus.
Indications	hip pain, sciatica, low back pain, two hip weakness, foot numbness.

50. Knee

Position	located in the depression, which is formed by the fifth toe and the leading edge of the calcaneus.
Indications	knee arthritis, knee pain, knee injuries, foot numbness.

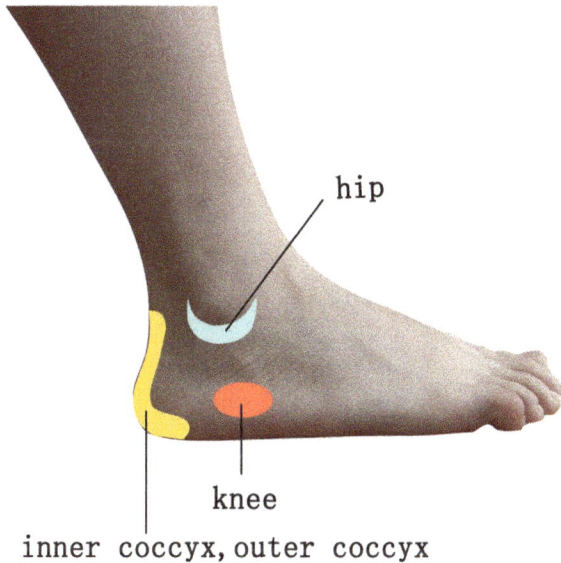

Figure 5-20 inner coccyx—knee

51. Elbow

Position	located at the bottom of the fifth metatarsal outside the feet, close to the metatarsal tuberosity.
Indications	elbow pain, elbow arthritis, elbow injuries, the sore arm, arm numbness.

52. Shoulder

Position	located at the fifth metatarsophalangeal.
Indications	frozen shoulder, arm pain, numbness in the hands of cataract.

53. Scapula

Position	located in the area shaped "Y" along the fourth and fifth toes to the cuboid of foot instep.
Indications	frozen shoulder, shoulder pain, shoulder movement disorder.

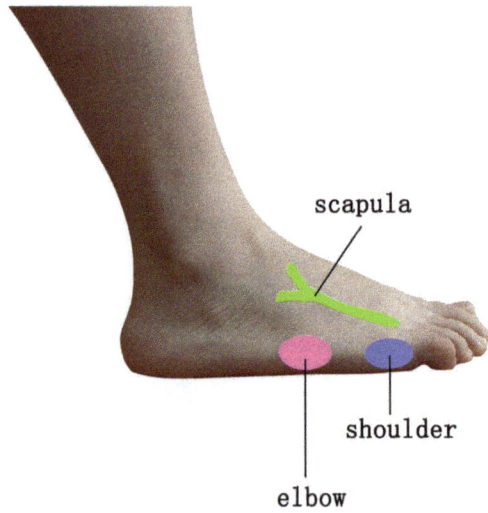

Figure 5-21 elbow—scapula

54. Throat and trachea

Position	located outside the first metatarsophalangeal joint of feet instep.
Indications	laryngitis, pharyngitis, cough, asthma, bronchitis, hoarseness, upper respiratory tract infection.

55. Chest (breast)

Position	located in the region formed by the middle part of the second, third and fourth metatarsal of feet instep.
Indications	chest pain, chest tightness, mastitis, breast hyperplasia, breast cancer, esophageal disease.

56. Ribs

Position	located in the feet instep, the region between the first cuneiform and the navicular is the inner ribs, the region between the third cuneiform and the cuboid is the outer ribs.
Indications	pleurisy, chest tightness, pleurisy, rib injury.

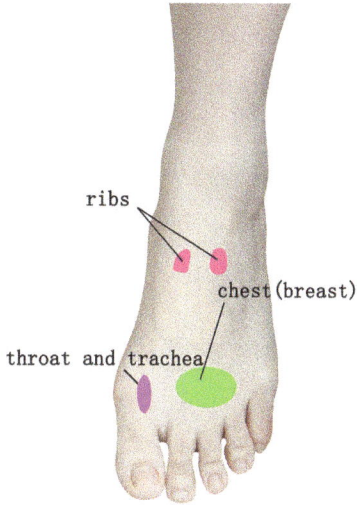

Figure 5-22 throat and trachea—ribs

57. Wrist

Position	located in the central depression of the navicular, cuboid and talar joints of feet instep.
Indications	Wrist pain, wrist arthritis, wrist injuries and hand numbness.

58. The labyrinth

Position	located at the leading edge of the sutura between the fourth and fifth toes of feet instep.
Indications	motion sickness, motion sickness, balance disorders, dizziness, vertigo, tinnitus, coma, high blood pressure, low blood pressure.

59. Maxillary and mandibular

Position	located on the feet instep, the front of the stripes of the interphalangeal of the thumb is the maxillary, the rear is the mandibular.
Indications	toothache, dental bleeding, gingivitis, mouth ulcers, snoring, and taste disturbance.

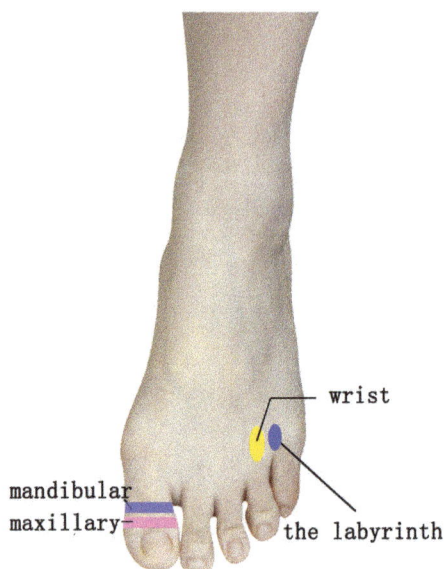

Figure 5-23 wrist—maxillary and mandibular

60. Tonsil

Position	located above the Section II of the feet instep, the both sides of the tendon.
Indications	tonsillitis, upper respiratory tract infections.

61. Chest lymph nodes

Position	located in the place between the first and second metatarsal of feet instep.
Indications	fever, inflammation, cysts, and enhance immunity of cancer.

62. Cervical lymph nodes

Position	located at the toes webbed of insteps and soles of feet.
Indications	cervical lymph node enlargement, goiter, hyperthyroidism, and toothache.

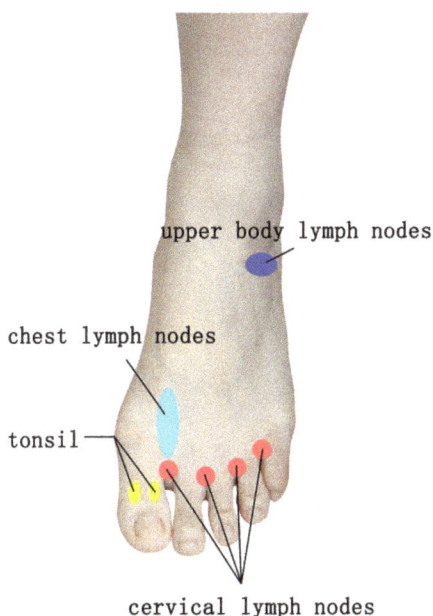

upper body lymph nodes

chest lymph nodes

tonsil

cervical lymph nodes

Figure 5-24 chest lymph nodes—upper body lymph nodes

63. Upper body lymph nodes

Position	located in the front of the ankle outside the feet instep, the depression which is formed by the talus and the lateral malleolus.
Indications	fever, inflammation, and cysts. Can enhance the immune anti-cancer ability.

64. Lower body lymph nodes

Position	located in the front of the ankle inside the feet instep, the depression which is formed by the talus and the medial malleolus.
Indications	fever, inflammation, and cysts.

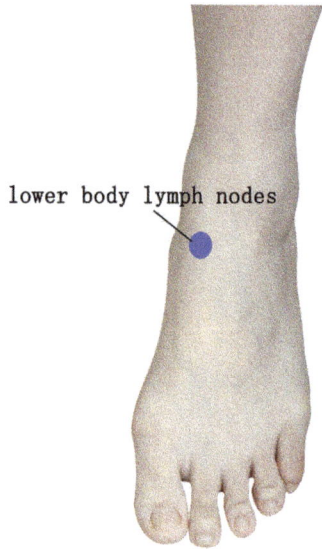

lower body lymph nodes

Figure 5-25 lower body lymph nodes

Wrist-ankle acupuncture

Wrist-ankle acupuncture (WAA) is a recently developed acupuncture therapy, in which needles are inserted just through the skin, and then advanced subcutaneously on the wrist, and the ankle, to treat various common diseases of the corresponding zones of the body where the symptoms and signs are located. Zones classification of clinical manifestation into six longitudinal zones, and set six entry points at the wrist and ankle. The body at the diaphragm is divided into upper and lower parts; selection of points on the basis of the longitudinal zones where the diseases is located. This method to treat aliments by using subcutaneous needling does not induce sensations of soreness, numbness, distension, heaviness or pain.

Divisions and Indications

WAA treatment divides the body into 6 parts, and most diseases can be classified as 6 longitudinal zones on both sides of the body as the points can be accurately located for the required part of the body. These zones are arranged along the longitudinal axis of the body, and be divided by anterior and inferior midlines. Divisions and indications of each zone are as follows:

Zone 1:	The longitudinal area along the anterior midline of the body, including the forehead, eyes, nose, tongue, trachea, lips, anterior teeth, throat, esophagus, heart, heart, abdomen, umbilicus, lower abdomen and perineum.
Indications	frontal headache, eye disease, nasal congestion, drooling, frontal toothache, sore throat, bronchitis, stomach pain, palpitations, biliary, enuresis, dysmenorrhea, vaginal discharge, etc.

Zone 2:	The longitudinal area on the anterior aspect of the body, including the ankle, cheeks, posterior teeth, lower jaw, thyroid, supraclavicular fossa, breast, lung, liver, gallbladder (right) and lateral abdomen.
Indications	anterotemporal headache, posterior toothache, distending pain of breast, chest pain, asthma, liver pain, pain in the chest and hypochondriac region.

Zone 3:	The exterior area on the anterior aspect of the body, covering a narrow vertical area along the anterior border of the ear and the anterior border of the axilla on the chest and abdomen.
Indications	less disease occurs in Zone 3, including temporal-auricular headache, chest pain or abdominal pain along the anterior border of the palate, etc.

Zone 4:	the area between the anterior and posterior aspects of the body. Covering the area from the vertex down to the ear lobe, and the trapezius of the shoulder. Covering the vertical area from the mid-axilla on the chest and abdomen down to the anterior superior iliac spine.
Indications	headache at vertex, tinnitus, deafness, dislocation of the mandibular joint, chest and abdominal pain below the armpit, etc.

Zone 5:	the longitudinal area on the posterolateral aspect of the trunk, just opposite to Zone 2, including the posterior part of the head, the posterolateral part of the neck, and the area along the scapular line passing down to the lumbar region.
Indications	posterotemporal head pain, stiff neck, pain in the scapular, lumbar vertebrae transverse process syndrome.

Zone 6:	the longitudinal area on the posterior midline of the trunk, just opposite to Zone 1, including the posterior head, the occipital part, the spinous process of the spine and the paravertebral, the appendix and the anus, etc.
Indications	occipital headache, pain in the area of cervical and thoracic vertebrae, acute lumbar sprain, lumbar muscle strain and so on, etc.

These 6 zones can be summarised as: distributed along the sides of the midline: Zone 1 in the front of the body, and Zone 6 in the back of the body. Distributed on the longitudinal area: Zone 2 in the front of the body, Zone 5 in the back of the body. Distributed at the front and rear junctions: Zone 4. Distributed on the front outer edge: Zone 3.

Centering on the junction of the sternum end and the rib arches on both sides, draw a horizontal line around the body representing the diaphragm. The horizontal line divides the six sides of the body into upper and lower zones. The areas above the horizontal line are called: Upper 1, Upper 2, Upper 3, Upper 4, Upper 5, Upper 6. The areas below the horizontal line are called: Lower 1, Lower 2, Lower 3, Lower 4, Lower 5, Lower 6.

To indicate the symptoms on the left or right side, it can be recorded as the UR1 (Upper right 1) or the LF6 (lower left 6).

For the extremities, when the upper and lower extremities are in the forward side of the inner side and the sides are close to each other, the inner side of the limb is equivalent to the front of the body; the outer side is equivalent to the back of the body; the first slit is equivalent to the front midline; the latter slit is equivalent to the posterior midline, so that the division of the limbs is similar to the body.

First find out the body area where the disease is located, and then selecting the insertion point in the same area on the wrist and ankle. There are 6 needle points in the wrist and ankle, each of which is consistent with the upper and lower 6 areas of the body, so each point can treat the disease in the body area consistent with it.

Positions and indications of the needle points

Part I The Needle Points of the Wrist

There are 6 needle points around the wrist, that form a circle on the 2 fingers, from the main horizontal, over the wrist stripes. From the ulnar side to the radial side of the palmar surface, to the radial side to the ulnar side of the doral surface, there are upper 1, upper 2, upper 3, upper 4, upper 5, and upper 6 orderly.

1. Upper 1

Position	between the ulnar side of the little finger and the ulnar wrist flexor tendon close to the depression of the inside of the tendon.
Indications	front headache, eye and nose diseases, trigeminal neuralgia, facial swelling, anterior teeth swelling, dizziness, sore throat, bronchitis, stomach pain, heart disease, hypertension, night sweats, chills, insomnia, rickets, etc.

2. Upper 2

Position	between the longus tendon and the iliac crest tendon in the center of the carpal-palm equivalent to Neiguan (PC 6) of the pericardium meridian.
Indications	anterotemporal headache, posterior toothache, submandibular pain and swelling, fullness in the chest, chest pain, asthma, pain in the center of the palm (the needle tip punctures upward), numbness of fingers (the needle tip punctures downward), etc.

3. Upper 3

Position	located on dorsal wrist triples on the 2-inches close to the edge of the radius, and lateral to the radial artery.
Indications	hypertension, chest pain.

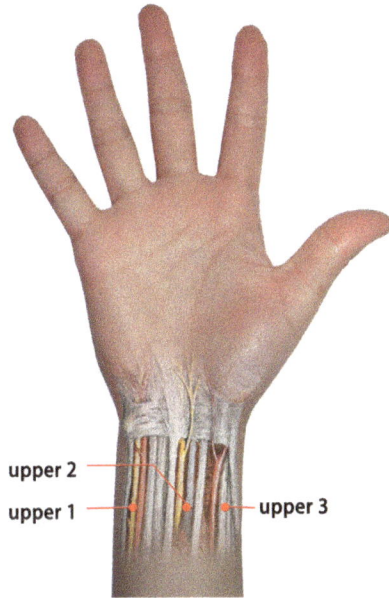

Figure 6-1 upper1—upper3

4. Upper 4

Position	in the radical side of the thumb with the patient's palm facing inward.
Indications	vertical headache, ear disease, temporomandibular joint disorders, pain at the anterior aspect of the shoulder, chest pain (along the mid-axillary line), etc.

5. Upper 5

Position	at the midpoint of the dorsal side of the wrist equivalent to Waiguan (TE 5) of the triple energizer meridian.
Indications	pain of posterior temples, sensory and motor impairment of upper limbs, joint pain of elbow, wrist and finger (the needle tip punctures downward), etc.

6. Upper 6

Position	on the ulnar side of the little finger
Indications	occipital headache, pains of nape, pain along the cervical vertebrae and the thoracic vertebrae, etc.

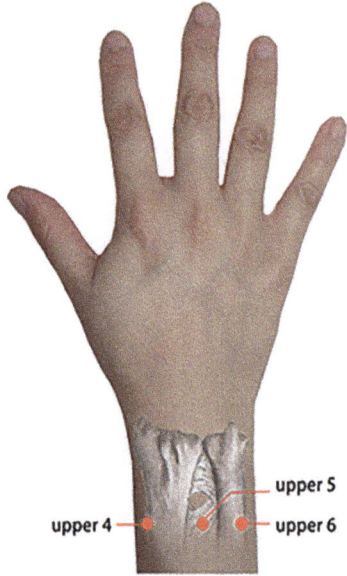

Figure 6-2 upper4-upper6

Part II The Needle Points of the Ankle

There are 6 points in ankle needle points, it is located at the top of the highest point of the inner and outer rafts upward the three horizontal fingers (equivalent to the lower end of the xuanzhong, Gb 39 and the Sanyinjiao, SP 6), from the inside of the Achilles tendon to the outer achilles tendon around a circle, followed by the Lower 1, Lower 2, Lower 3, Lower 4, Lower 5, Lower 6.

1. Lower 1

Position	on the inner edge of the Achilles tendon.
Indications	epigastric distention and pain, pain around the navel, dysmenorrhea, leukorrhagia, enuresis, genital itching, heel pain (the tip of the needle is facing downward).

2. Lower 2

Position	near the posterior border of the tibia bone in the center of the medial aspect.
Indications	pain over the liver, pain of the side abdominal, allergic enteritis, etc.

3. Lower 3

Position	1cm medical to the anterior border of the tibia bone.
Indications	knee (inner edge) joint pain, etc.

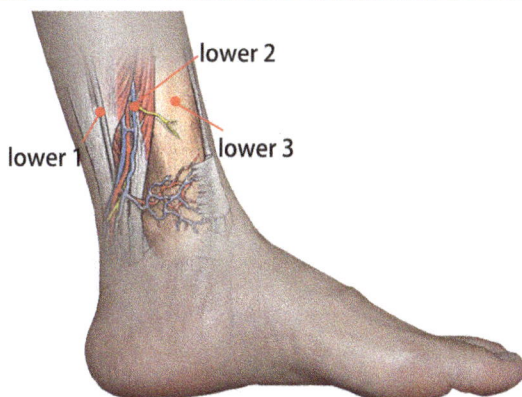

Figure 6-3 lower1-lower3

4. Lower 4

Position	at the midpoint between the anterior border of the fibula and the anterior border of the tibia.
Indications	pain of quadriceps femoris, pain of knee joint, lower limb sensory disturbance (numbness, allergies), lower extremity dyskinesia (sputum, limb fibrillation, chorea), pain of phalangeal joint (the needle tip punctures downward), etc.

5. Lower 5

Position	the center of the lateral side near the posterior border of the fibula.
Indications	pain of hip joint, ankle sprain (joint) (the needle tip punctures downward), etc.

6. Lower 6

Position	near the lateral border of tendon calcaneus.
Indications	treating diseases located in the Lower 6. Such as acute lumbar sprain, lumbar muscle strain, pain of sacroiliac articulation, sciatica, pain of gastrocnemius muscle, dorsal digital pain of foot (the needle tip punctures downward), etc,.

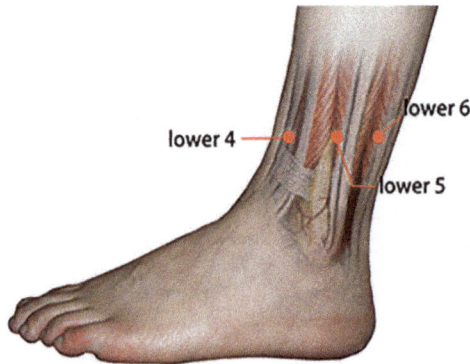

Figure 6-4 lower4-lower6

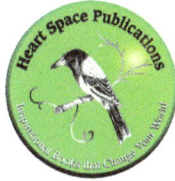

If you derived benefit from this manual,
please see the other three in the series

Quick Reference Handbooks of Chinese Medicine

Acupuncture of Acupoint Combinations Quick Lookups

Illustrations of Special Effective Acupoints for common
Diseases

Human Body Reflex Zone Quick Lookup,
Bilingual anatomical illustration of reflex zones
(English edition)

Quick Investigation On Acupunture Points – Selection of
Professor Yang Jiasan

Go to www.heartspacepublications.com